Mediterranean Diet for Beginners

A Straightforward Guide Outlining Simple Rules for Weight Loss and a 2-Week Meal Plan to Get You Started

Jenna Andrews

Table of Contents

Introduction

The world at large, but especially the Western countries, often have the idea that being on a diet involves restricting ourselves. This has become so common to the point that it has greatly increased the number of people suffering from malnourishment, dehydration, hunger, and eating disorders. However, just because you are on a diet doesn't mean you are necessarily dieting. While dieting involves going from one method of restrictive eating to the next, "diet" simply refers to what you eat. Some people may have healthy diets, while others choose to eat cheeseburgers, fries, and soda on a daily basis. Part of the reason for this is that many Americans have never been well-taught about what constitutes a healthy diet.

In this book, you will learn about what is frequently claimed to be one of the healthiest diets around—the Mediterranean diet. These claims are not only promoted by some of the biggest names in medicine such as the Mayo Clinic; they are also backed by years of well-established research. You don't have to deprive yourself or become unhealthy to lose weight. You can attain the weight loss you desire and remain healthy all on the same eating style. With the Mediterranean diet, originating from the natural diets of people in Greece and Italy, you can enjoy a number of ingredients such as vegetables, whole grains, legumes, nuts, seafood, olive oil, and even red wine!

Eating this way has been shown to not only increase weight loss but also reduce the risk of disease and increase lifespans. Scientists have thoroughly researched how these ingredients independently and co-dependently are able to improve people's lives for the better. Eating this way, you will enjoy delicious meals and increased energy—all while enjoying a glass of red wine.

If this all sounds too good to be true, don't worry. All of these benefits and many more will be well-examined clearly and conversationally within this book. You no longer have to switch from one unhealthy diet to the next. Instead, make the choice to improve your life with a healthy and delicious diet that has been enjoyed for centuries and researched for decades.

With this book, you will be provided with all of the tools you need to succeed. All you have to do is start.

Chapter 1

The Mediterranean Diet – A Historical Approach

Simply put, the Mediterranean diet consists of eating healthy monosaturated fats such as those found in olive oil and avocados, rather than saturated fats found in meat or coconut oil. Along with these healthy fats, people eat a high number of plant-based foods such as whole grains, vegetables, fruits, legumes, nuts, and seeds; a moderate or high number of fish and shellfish; a low number of animal-based products, such as meat and dairy; and lastly, what many people enjoy, a daily glass of red wine. Of course, if you are underage, struggle with addiction, are on medication, or have another reason you are unable to or prefer not to drink wine—that is okay as well. However, red wine and the other foods on the Mediterranean diet have many benefits to your weight loss, health, and well-being.

However, many people may wonder how this style of eating came about. The Mediterranean diet was created naturally by observing the eating habits of people within Mediterranean countries such as Greece, Italy, Lebanon, and some others. The people in these countries simply consume what is native to their land and that which grows well. While the ingredients enjoyed in the Mediterranean may be everyday foods, especially to those who live there, they are packed with powerful nutrients that can powerfully affect a person's life when consumed regularly.

The climate of the Mediterranean is rather unique. This geographical location is often referred to as "the cradle of society" by historians. This is because, in the Mediterranean, the entire history of the ancient world occurred. The ancient civilizations of the Babylonians, Sumerians, Persians, and Assyrians took place in here. The ancient powers of the Cretans, Phoenicians, Greeks, and Romans grew overtime within these regions. You will even find the banks of the great Nile river along the Mediterranean. These areas became vital in society, as they became a meeting place for cultures to grow and develop, people to meet, religions to deepen, languages to grow, customs to be adopted, and entire lifestyles to be changed. It is impossible to overstate how important the Mediterranean cultures were to world history and development.

This rich and intricate history and development is what lead to what we now know as the Mediterranean diet. While we don't know when the roots of this diet first took place, anthropologists have been able to learn how different cultures grew and developed from their contact with one another to further adopt this eating style. These anthropologists have been able to date the Mediterranean diet back to the Middle Ages when the Roman Empire adopted some eating styles from the Greek.

The Romans based much of their diet—and even part of their faith—on bread, oils, and wine. These primary components of their diets were consumed with large quantities of fish and seafood, which were quite prevalent in Roman society due to their freshness. The elite Romans especially enjoyed fried and grilled fish, along with fried or raw oysters. To supplement these ingredients, the Romans would also partake in vegetables such as lettuce, mushrooms, leeks, chicory, mallow, as well as a small amount of sheep's cheese.

However, the fare of slaves within the Roman empire was obviously much more restricted. These people would consume large amounts of bread, along with half a pound of olives, olive oil, and some salted fish. These people were rarely able to consume meat or cheese.

The dietary customs of the Roman empire continued to develop as they interacted with Germanic nomads nearby. These nomads lived closely in harmony with nature by gathering food, gardening, and hunting. The Germanic nomads would raise pigs for their fat content, grow vegetables, and even grow some grain. However, this grain was not used to produce bread as it would be by the Romans, but rather to ferment into beer.

The Romans and nomads would adopt some of the other cultures' eating habits, but overall, the Roman Empire was unwilling to change its Mediterranean diet for that of the nomad's. However, the Mediterranean aspects of bread, oil, and wine was partially adopted, which lead to it soon being exported and partially adopted within the European regions. Before long, this trilogy of bread, oil, and wine would become central elements within the Christian religion and used to feed the middle and lower class people within Europe. The combination of the food cultures from the Christian Roman Empire and the Germanic people would over time lead to the development of a new culture in food, that of the Arabs located on the southern side of the Mediterranean.

The Arabs soon influenced the agricultural and plant-based ingredients commonly used within the Mediterranean diet. While most of these ingredients, such as eggplant, spinach, citrus, sugar, cane, and spices were only used by the wealthy, they would become more commonplace over time.

The discovery of America would later impact the foods used within the Mediterranean, as well. With this discovery, the Mediterranean was soon introduced to tomatoes, potatoes, corn, beans, chilies, and peppers. The tomato had only recently been discovered to be edible and was therefore considered exotic and exciting. This red fruit would soon become a large part of the Mediterranean diet, going so far as to be considered a symbol of their cuisine.

While vegetables became an integral element of the Mediterranean diet, grains and cereals maintained their spot as one of the three elements of the Mediterranean, along with oils and wine. This is primarily because grains and cereals are simple to store for long periods and easy to cook. Importantly, these grains and cereals would also limit hunger pangs of the lower and middle classes, allowing them to work through their days. The specific grains and cereals these people consumed varied based on their location within the Mediterranean, but bread, pasta, polenta, couscous, and soups with grains within them were all common features.

As you can see, the Mediterranean diet consists of many cultures coming together to form one of the optimal cuisines for health, wellness, and longevity. From the formation of the Roman empire to the discovery of America, the Mediterranean diet is comprised of many well-rounded and health-promoting components. Submitted to UNESCO, the Candidature Dossier fully defines the Mediterranean diet as being a social practice which contains the components of fishing, harvesting, processing, preparation, conservation, and cooking in such as used by various cultures within the Mediterranean Basin. This is a simple cuisine, yet full of nutrition and flavor.

This cuisine has persevered over the centuries due to its massive health benefits. The Mediterranean diet has been found to treat obesity, diabetes, high blood pressure, and more.

While the Mediterranean diet may still be relatively new to America and other non-Mediterranean countries, there are twenty-two countries that have been benefiting from this way of eating for an exceptionally long time. During the early 1600s, some people from the Mediterranean even began to attempt to share these health benefits with other countries. After seeing how few plant-based ingredients the British consumed in 1614, the Italian Giacomo Castelvetro published the book A Brief Account of the Fruits, Herbs, and Vegetables of Italy.

While living in England after being exiled from Italy he was horrified by the state of the English's diet and felt the need to help increase the nutrition of those around him. Not only did he attempt to encourage the English to consume an increasing number of plant-based foods, but he also exhorted the benefits of preparing these ingredients in specific ways. He hoped that this would both increase their health and the flavor of their food. The book he published contains beneficial ingredients, gardening tips, advice for how to keep cooking hygienic, and delicious recipes. Castelvetro passionately wrote his book, even going so far as to emotionally write about how to properly prepare a salad with a mixture of fresh herbs, tender lettuce, olive oil, and vinegar. While some people may see a salad as a bland and boring food, the way that Castelvetro prepared and wrote about salads is far from bland or boring—rather, you can practically taste all of the flavors as he describes the vivacious and fresh ingredients to make use of. Castelvetro was far from talking about food in a bland medical fashion, instead, he believed that the taste should be as important as the health benefits. This belief is still applicable today when we don't want to simply eat to live but to instead enjoy both a full and delicious life. Nobody is likely to stick to a bland and boring diet, nor should we have to.

Sadly, despite the English's adoption of Italian fashion, architecture, language, and gardens, they were less keen on adopting the dietary lifestyle. The English had concurred many countries, yet decided to keep their foods relatively the same over time. Because of this, few were willing to take up the recommendations of Castelvetro.

During the 1950s and 1960s a researcher, Dr. Ancel Keys, found that people on the large Grecian island of Crete experienced increased health and longevity. Dr. Keys' hypothesis was that this increase in health was due to the natural wonders grown on the island that the people at on a regular basis. The difference of healthy within America and Crete was so astounding that the rates of death from heart disease and cancer within America prior to World War II were nearly three times higher than the death rates in Crete. During the time of Dr. Keys' interest, the island of Crete was still not affected by the rise in processed and fast foods that occurred widely after World War II, making it an ideal place to study the eating habits.

However, this is the simplified version. There are much more history and research that have gone into what is widely known as one of the healthiest lifestyles. This research is important to know if you hope to fully understand the benefits this eating style offers. Let's take a journey through the past to find how we can better live in the present.

Firstly, how did Dr. Ancel Keys discover the benefits of the Mediterranean diet? While the people living in the Mediterranean and therefore naturally eating this way were aware to an extent of the benefits, prior to this point in time there had been no studies comparing the Mediterranean diet to other common diets and lifestyles. The reason that Dr. Keys was able to make this discovery was caused in large part by the Italian-Americans who had settled down within New York. After looking at the lives of these Italian Americans Dr. Keys noticed that even the wealthy citizens within New York were having more illness struggles and overall poor health than the poor citizens within southern Italy. After examining the differences in these people's lifestyles, Dr. Keys hypothesized that the difference was due to food and the ingredients that made up their diets.

This hypothesis led Dr. Keys to conduct a famous study, known as the Seven Countries Study taking place in the United States, Italy, Greece, Yugoslavia, Finland, Holland, and Japan. The purpose of this study was to research the connection between nutrition, lifestyles, and cardiovascular diseases within different countries and regions. Dr. Keys hypothesized that this study would prove the nutritional value of the Mediterranean diet and how it could improve many people's lives for the better while lowering their risk of disease.

The study conducted by Dr. Keys revealed that the people on a natural Mediterranean diet presented with surprisingly low levels of cholesterol and an extremely low risk of cardiovascular diseases. The results were found to be due to the high number of bread, pasta, vegetables, spices, herbs, and olive oil within their diet, along with the minimal use of meat products.

Within the published paper on the Seven Countries Study, Dr. Keys explained how within the Mediterranean a diet people commonly eat pasta with tomato sauce and a touch of Parmesan, homemade minestrone soup, fresh fish, bread straight from the oven, beans and vegetables drizzled with olive oil, fruit for dessert, with only a minimal amount of meat.

After Dr. Key's research was published it led to the development of many more scientific studies on the Mediterranean diet and its benefits for chronic disease and overall health. Overall, most people were able to agree that the Mediterranean diet is one of the healthiest and natural ways of eating, calling for moderation of healthy foods rather than the elimination of entire food groups. This was widely shown in studies which found that by switching a person's lifestyle to fit that of a Mediterranean diet they can greatly decrease abdominal fat, lower blood glucose levels, decrease blood triglycerides, increase the healthy HDL cholesterol, and lower high blood pressure.

However, it's important to note that simply switching to the Mediterranean diet alone may not improve your heart health. You are not always able to gain the health you seek if you change one aspect of your life if the other portions of your life are still detrimental. If you never exercise, eat a large increase in calories, smoke, have high-stress levels, or do drugs then you are still likely to develop many chronic diseases, including cardiovascular diseases. After all, studies have found that half of the reported strokes have occurred in people who have low levels of blood cholesterol. Dr. Ancel Keys stressed the importance of not only adopting the Mediterranean diet but an overall healthy lifestyle if you hope to increase your health and longevity.

While the Mediterranean diet may be a balanced and natural diet, more people have not taken it up as society slowly pushes toward foods enjoyed by the affluent or to those promoted within crash diets. This leads to people avoiding beans while promoting steaks. Disregarding potatoes and leaning toward sugary desserts. People choose low-carbohydrate or low-fat rather than a balanced number of these nutrients from healthy sources.

The rise in fad diets that would for a long time prevent many Americans from seeing the benefits of a balanced Mediterranean lifestyle began largely in the late nineteenth and early twentieth centuries. During this time period, there were many dubious dietary claims made, with the people promoting them claiming them as beneficial. This largely took place as Americans attempted to change the dietary of the poor and immigrants who had recently settled into the country. Social workers, economists, and nurses believed that they could change the very nature of immigrants and lower class people by changing their dietary habits.

The faux food "science" of this era led people to believe that foreign eating habits were unhealthy and uneconomical. People began to believe that these foods were overly difficult to digest, over-seasoned leading to stomach disorders, and could somehow lead to alcoholism. Society grasped hold of this pseudoscience, believing that garlic (which is common on the Mediterranean diet) was the enemy and should be avoided at all cost. People largely avoided fresh fruits and vegetables, believing that they were primarily full of water and therefore void of nutritional benefits. The health-promoting bran on grains and skin on potatoes was disregarded, meanwhile, highly processed white flour was promoted.

However, the reformers of America's dietary habits soon gave up on changing the habits of immigrants. The immigrants had resisted the change and instead chose to continue enjoying the food of their homelands. This was for their benefit, as the reformers only brought about negative changes for the middle class by fooling them with convincing pseudoscience. By the beginning of the twentieth century, this pseudoscience and food faddism had taken over America, completely changing dietary habits for years to come.

While the dietary habits of Americans may be different now than they were at the beginning of the twentieth century, pseudoscience still heavily promotes food fads, leading to misinformation, damaged metabolism, eating disorders, malnutrition, and weight which yo-yos back and forth for many individuals.

The natural order of human food intake has been interrupted by this change, as well. Historically, anthropologists Sidney Mintz has explained that humans have gone through two important food revolutions which changed the way we eat worldwide. The first of these revolutions was when we first began to domesticate animals and plants through farming, allowing humans for the first time to take control over our food supply, what we eat, how much we eat, and when we eat.

The second human food revolution occurred when processed sugars and fats began to alter the human diet. Throughout most of history, we ate mainly complex carbohydrate (such as grains) with the addition of legumes, a small amount of other protein, and olive oil. You can see examples of this in many cultures, such as rice and beans eaten in Asia, tortillas, and beans in Mexico, black bread and cheese in Russia, and more. However, this natural and healthy balanced nutrition was disrupted when we began to consume soft drinks in place of water. In fact, in many communities, these sugar-filled and artificial sweetener-filled soft drinks have replaced water as the most consumed beverage.

People of all ages choose to eat potato chips, ice cream, cake, muffins, doughnuts, fried chicken, and double-decker bacon cheeseburgers in place of the nutritionally balanced fare of our ancestors. However, when people begin to gain weight from this heavily processed diet they often switch to weight loss diets which only set them up for failure. There are a number of these diets but many of them cause a person to avoid important nutrients such as grains or olive oil, eat much less than their bodies require, and may even only allow a small amount of bland boring food. These diets, while sometimes recommended by doctors, are in fact incredibly unhealthy. The truth is that doctors regularly are not given very much education on what constitutes a healthy diet.

Although, if you talk with a nutritionist or dietitian who has studied heavily on the subject, they will recommend a balanced and healthy lifestyle that doesn't eliminate food groups, such as the Mediterranean diet.

While a crash or fad diet may help you to see results more quickly than a more balanced diet, this is an unhealthy type of weight loss. The weight loss brought about by these diets causes the body to go into a state of metabolic dysfunction, often causing a person to quickly regain weight after quitting the unmaintainable diet. This not only causes stress and frustration to the person as they find the pounds piling back on, but it is poor for their health and can increase the risk of developing dangerous diseases later down the road. The Mediterranean diet may take a little more time to result in the desired amount of weight loss, but this is beneficial as you can lose weight at a more maintainable speed, increasing your health and likelihood of keeping the pounds at bay. You don't want to go on a diet only to regain the weight, it is better to choose a healthy lifestyle which will keep you happy, healthy, and at your desired weight long down the road in the future.

In conclusion, while the Mediterranean diet may promote limiting meat and dairy products, unlike many crash and fad diets, it doesn't promote eliminating entire food groups. On the contrary, the Mediterranean lifestyle promotes balancing the necessary nutrients required to not only sustain life but to help the mind and body thrive. As the Mediterranean is a geographical location full of nutrient-dense ingredients with all of the components humans require for survival this lifestyle developed naturally over time, proving its maintainability and many health benefits.

While fad and crash diets are still all the rage every January and summer as people look to lose weight after the holidays and before going to the beach, there is simply no need for a diet which will only cause you more problems in the long-run. Instead, if you choose to enjoy a full Mediterranean lifestyle you will find you can enjoy all your favorite foods in moderation while being sustained with whole grains, legumes, fruits, vegetables, fish, seafood, olive oil, and wine on a day-to-day basis. This will increase your health while decreasing your weight. The Mediterranean lifestyle is full of rich traditions which can tempt your pallet and keep you satisfied time and time again as you enjoy the full range of flavors it has to offer.

Chapter 2
The Science Behind the Mediterranean Diet and Why It Works

The scientific effects of the Mediterranean diet have been researched ever since Dr. Ancel Keys first conducted his *Seven Countries Study*. It's important to keep in mind that during the modern age, the Mediterranean diet has changed from its healthy natural balance to include unhealthier fast foods and junk foods. Therefore, when studies on the Mediterranean diet are conducted, it is specifically referencing their diet prior to 1960.

The Mediterranean diet during the early 1960s includes an abundance of vegetables, legumes, fruits, whole grains and other cereals, nuts, and seeds. Sugar and honey are eaten minimally, with fruit usually serving as a dessert. The main source of fat is olive oil, with the addition of some fish and seafood. Wine is served in low to moderate amounts, usually on a daily basis with meals. Meats, eggs, dairy products, and saturated fats are eaten in minimal amounts.

Previous data show that during this period the people of Crete, Greece were physically active by working in the kitchen and fields—resulting in a much lower rate of obesity than that within America and Northern Europe. Similarly, the life expectancy of adults was among the highest within the world, with extremely low rates of cancer, chronic diseases, and cardiovascular diseases.

There have been multiple studies and consensuses on the Mediterranean diet. A 1998 statement of consensus found that diets which are high in vegetables, fruits, legumes, and whole grains are especially helpful. These diets may also include fish, low-fat dairy, and nuts. While some people may be concerned about the fat level, the researchers found that as long as calories are not eaten in excess then the fat within this diet does not need to be restricted as long as it is from healthy sources. This diet is beneficial because it contains a large number of healthy fats while largely excluding saturated fats and hydrogenated or partially hydrogenated fats.

There is another consensus from the year 2000 discussing the fat within the Mediterranean diet and the benefits it has in health and longevity. This consensus found that there are a large number and an increasing amount of scientific evidence proving the benefits of the Mediterranean diet. Similar to the 1998 consensus, the 2000 consensus found that diets high in the previously mentioned food groups and olive oil are beneficial to overall human health. This consensus also found that there is no need to limit the number of healthy fats you are eating from olives and fish, as long as you are eating the correct number of calories for your body type.

The World Health Organization, also known as W.H.O, concluded that the Mediterranean diet is an effective approach to preventing and controlling non-contractible diseases. These diseases are the leading causes of premature death of people under the age of sixty-five years old, and by controlling these causes of death we can greatly increase the population's general lifespan and health. While some diets that may help treat diseases and common causes of premature death are difficult to follow, that is not true of the Mediterranean lifestyle. This diet is extremely simple and easy to follow, so much so in fact that the World Health Organization rated it as the number one easiest-to-follow diet. Following the Mediterranean diet in ease were Weight Watchers and the Flexitarian diet. However, these two choices did not compare with respect to their effectiveness and health benefits. By being the simplest to follow and user-friendly diet people are much more likely to stick to it and therefore receive the benefits.

It's easy to say a diet has many benefits, it's another thing to have the science to back it up. Within the remainder of this chapter, we will look at some of the most compelling science which backs up the Mediterranean diet, proving its many health benefits.

Behind the Fats

We all know that there are both good and bad fats. However, many people are unaware of which fats are quantified as "bad" and which are "good." Why are some fats good for us while others are harmful? In order to understand the Mediterranean diet, it's important to understand the types of fats it promotes, and how these fats promote our overall health and longevity.

Rather than forsaking all fat and removing it from our diet no matter the source we should promote the use of healthy fats. These healthy fats are a wonderful source of energy for the body which promotes the growth of cell membranes, protects out nervous system, forms the exterior of many cells, and promotes the absorption of many vitamins and minerals. Not only that, but fat is essential to control our body's inflammation response, proper blood clotting when we develop injuries and cuts to prevent excessive bleeding and to influence the movement of our muscles.

While all fats molecules have a similar fatty acid molecular structure, they may have different effects on the body. Each fat molecule contains hydrogen atoms which are attached to a chain of carbon atoms. However, not all fat molecules look the same. Some of these molecules have a longer or differently shaped chain of carbon molecules or a different number of hydrogen atoms. These differences may seem trivial, but the molecular difference causes these fats to interact with our bodies in various ways.

Saturated Fats

The In-Between Fats

One of the most common fats within the American diet is saturated fats. Some of them are better than others, depending on their source. Generally, they are neither helpful or detrimental.

Saturated fats are called thus due to the number of hydrogen atoms that surround each of the carbon atoms. In fact, each carbon atom is surrounded with as many hydrogen atoms as is possible. Saturated fats such as coconut oil, bacon grease, and others, are able to stay solid when they are at room temperature rather than being suspended in a liquid state. Prominent sources of saturated fats include red meat, coconut oil, dairy products, and baked goods which have been commercially prepared.

There are some saturated fats that are better than others. For instance, coconut oil has more benefits than the fat found within red meat. However, despite coconut oil's many benefits, saturated fats are not an optimal choice in large number. These fats increase cholesterol, causing us to have more harmful cholesterol (LDL) and less good cholesterol (HDL). This increase in bad cholesterol can lead to blockages within our bodies, even within the arteries surrounding the human heart!

In general, nutritionists recommend that we consume no more than ten percent of our daily caloric intake from sources of saturated fat.

Trans Fats

The Harmful Fat

The most damaging type of fat is trans fats. These fats have been altered with the hydrogenation process, which transmutes healthy oils into solid fat. This process not only makes the fats an easier consistency to work with, but it also prevents them from spoiling by going rancid. While this process may be beneficial for giant corporations who want to save money on ingredients that won't spoil, the hydrogenation process removes all health benefits from the oil and are completely damaging to the body. The fats are so harmful to the body to the point that they contain no benefits and have officially been banned within America.

However, while hydrogenated trans fats may be banned within America now, for a time they were incredibly prevalent. During the nineteen-hundreds, these fats were found in large concentration in vegetable shortening and margarine. Companies continued to find new ways to utilize these fats later in the century, using hydrogenated vegetable oils in fast food and commercially-prepared baked goods.

By eating trans fats the number of damaging LDL cholesterol in the bloodstream is increased while the helpful HDL cholesterol is lowered. The intake of trans fats has been directly linked to increased inflammation, cardiovascular disease, diabetes, stroke, insulin resistance, and other chronic illnesses. While saturated fats may be okay in moderation, even a small number of trans fats causes direct harm to the body. For each two percent of daily calories you eat from trans fats in a day your risk of heart disease increases by a whopping twenty-three percent!

Monounsaturated and Polyunsaturated Fats

The Good Fats

The best sources of fats frequently come from fish, vegetables, nuts, and seeds. These fat molecules have fewer hydrogen atoms than saturated fats, which ensures that they remain in their liquid state at room temperature. There are two main types of healthy fats, which are monounsaturated and polyunsaturated fats.

Polyunsaturated fats, like monounsaturated fats, are an incredibly beneficial type of fat. People use these fats quite frequently while cooking, as they are found in high number in sunflower, corn, and safflower oils. This is beneficial as polyunsaturated fats are essential for the human body, as they are vital for bodily functions yet we are unable to produce them on our own. These fats help manage inflammation, the healthy clotting of blood, muscle movement, and even build the cell membranes that protect out nerves and nervous system. These fats can also help lower the harmful LDL cholesterol, blood triglycerides, and overall cholesterol levels.

Polyunsaturated fats have two or more double bonds within the carbon chain. You will frequently hear of this with the two main types of polyunsaturated fats: omega-6 and omega-3 fatty acids. The number difference in these two types of fatty acid molecules refers to the exact distance between the beginning of the carbon chain and its first double bond within the molecule. While both types have benefits, it's important to have the correct ratio for optimal health. In the Western diet people typically have too many omega-6 fatty acids and too few omega-3 fatty acids. This is especially harmful to people with chronic illnesses, as too high of an omega-6 level can increase inflammation. A study on the importance of the omega-6 and omega-3 ratio on chronically ill patients found the ideal ratio was generally two to five parts omega-6 to one-part omega-3. The same study found that people who ate ten parts omega-6 to one-part omega-3 experienced negative side effects.

Omega-3 fatty acids can help lower inflammation, reduce high blood pressure, raise the beneficial HDL cholesterol, lower blood triglycerides, prevent potentially lethal heart arrhythmias, lower the risk of cardiovascular disease, and prevent stroke. Studies have even found that omega-3 fatty acids can prevent the need for corticosteroid medication for people living with rheumatoid arthritis.

Some excellent sources for omega-3 fatty acids include sardines, salmon, mackerel, walnuts, flaxseeds, canola oil, and non-hydrogenated soybean oil. Similarly, omega-6 fatty acids have been shown to lower the risk of cardiovascular disease when eaten in a healthy ratio with omega-3 fatty acids. You can find omega-6 in high number within soybean, safflower, sunflower, and corn oils as we as within walnuts.

On the Mediterranean lifestyle, you will be consuming most of your fats from olive oil, olives, and avocados. These ingredients are mainly comprised of monosaturated fats, which have a single carbon-to-carbon double bind. This means that monounsaturated fats have fewer hydrogen atoms than saturated fats and bend at their double bond. You will find that the structure of the monosaturated fats ensures that it remains liquid when at room temperature. Along with olives and avocados, other good sources of monounsaturated fat include canola oil, peanut oil, high-oleic sunflower, and safflower oils, and most nuts. Health experts and the Institute of Medicine recommend that the fats within our diet primarily source from monounsaturated and polyunsaturated fats. Not only did Dr. Keys oversee the famous Seven Countries Study which found the benefits of the Mediterranean diet, but through this process, he even helped to discover the very basis of the health benefits within monounsaturated fats.

There are different types of monounsaturated fats, but the most frequently occurring type is oleic acid. This type of fatty acid and monounsaturated fat composes approximately ninety percent of the monounsaturated fats within a person's diet. Other types of monounsaturated fats include vaccenic acid and palmitoleic acid. When consuming foods high in these fats, remember that ingredients rarely have a single source of fat—rather, they are comprised of a combination of multiple fats. For instance, while olive oil is approximately seventy-five percent monounsaturated fats (specifically oleic acid), there are a few other fats in there as well.

Oleic acid has many health benefits and is known as an omega-9 fatty acid. This type of fat when in pure form is often lacking in color and odor, although many of the products that contain it do have a yellowish tint and slight flavor. Olive and avocado oils are a wonderful example of this.

Oleic acid and therefore omega-9 fatty acids do not have a recommended daily serving, as they are found naturally within our cells. Due to our body producing the minimum amount of needed oleic acid it is sometimes considered a non-essential type of fatty acid to consume within our diets. However, study after study has found that people experience many benefits when supplementing their diets with oleic oil. After all, the oleic acid within olives is one of the founding principles of the Mediterranean diet which has shown many positive effects on people's lives.

One of the areas in which we can witness the positive effects of oleic acid is on our body's weight and fat. By replacing carbohydrates and other sources of fat with oleic acid many studies have shown that people can increase the burning of body fat and increase overall body weight and fat.

In a large comparison of twenty-four scientific studies, it was found that high-monounsaturated fat diets are more effective in weight loss than high-carbohydrate diets. This means that the Mediterranean diet, which replaces many sources of unhealthy calories with healthy monounsaturated fats, can great decrease fat and body weight.

However, oleic acid has more benefits than just weight loss, there are many other health benefits that can be achieved by increasing it within your diet. Another of the benefits you can achieve is a reduced risk of heart disease. This is especially true if you are replacing saturated fats, such as those from animals, with oleic acid. While a large amount of cholesterol within the bloodstream clogs arteries, leads to heart attacks, stroke, and heart disease, there are ways in which you can lower your risks of developing these problems or even directly confront them. Studies have shown that by increasing the oleic acid within your diet you can greatly reduce your risk of developing these conditions and lower your overall cholesterol level.

In one study, one-hundred and sixty-two people were observed as they completed a three month long high-monounsaturated fat diet along with a control group on a high-saturated fat diet. At the end of the study it found that while the high-saturated fat group experienced an increase by four percent in the unhealthy LDL cholesterol, the other group experienced quite different results. The high-monounsaturated group experienced a stunning five percent decrease in LDL cholesterol!

There are even more ways in which this simple fat can improve your heart health. I a study conducted on one-hundred and sixty-four patients diagnosed with high blood pressure found that eating a diet high in oleic acid and other monounsaturated fats lead to a significant decrease in blood pressure, as well as a lowered risk of heart disease. These improvements were markedly better than those received on a low-carbohydrate diet. Similar studies have found the same improvement in blood pressure in people with either metabolic syndrome or type II diabetes after consuming a high-monounsaturated fat diet.

Regarding diabetes, oleic acid can impact this dangerous disease, as well. It's important for our bodies to be able to properly produce insulin in order to prevent chronically high blood sugar and the resulting type II diabetes. Insulin is a vital hormone that controls our blood sugar and its movement. Being able to better control our insulin is important for not only preventing diabetes but improving the management and treatment in those who may already have the disease, as well. Studies have found that eating a diet high in oleic acid can improve the insulin response both in people with and without high blood sugar or diabetes.

In a study on nearly five-hundred people with metabolic syndrome, it was found that individuals on a high-monounsaturated fat diet for a period of twelve weeks were able to greatly reduce and manage insulin resistance. Insulin resistance leads to diabetes and increased weight, making treating this condition vital. In another study, it was found that after eating a diet high in oleic acid for three months one-hundred and sixty-two people were able to improve their insulin response by nine percent.

Inflammation is a healthy and important aspect of the human immune system when utilized correctly. The problem is that some people develop increased inflammation slowly over time. This increase of inflammation increases overall pain, infections, and even your likelihood of developing deadly diseases and illnesses. Some diets, such as the typical Western diet and those high in saturated fats, promote the increase in chronic inflammation. On the other hand, oleic acid and the Mediterranean diet have been shown to lower inflammation levels to that which is healthy.

In one study, it was found that people who consume a Mediterranean diet, which is naturally high in oleic acid, experienced a significant decrease in inflammation-related chemicals within their bloodstream. Another study found that people on a high-monounsaturated fat diet who have metabolic syndrome experienced a much greater decrease in inflammation than those on a high-saturated fat diet. Lastly, high-monounsaturated fat diets don't only reduce the inflammation chemicals within the bloodstream, but it can even reduce the inflammation genes held within fat tissue. This is one reason as to why these fats may aid in weight loss.

Cancer, one of the number one killers in the modern world, can even be impacted by oleic acid and other monounsaturated fats. Certain cancers, such as prostate and breast cancers, have specifically been found to be affected by an increase of monounsaturated fats in the diet. While more research is needed, some studies suggest that an increase in monounsaturated fats may protect against prostate cancer. A study conducted in Spain on six-hundred and forty-two women found that those who consume a higher amount of oleic acid, in turn, have lower rates of breast cancer. It has been suggested that olive oil may have some additional benefits in protecting against breast cancer, as people in Spain eat a much larger amount of this oil than people in many other countries. This can especially be promising for those on the Mediterranean diet, as the use of olive oil is an integral aspect of the lifestyle.

Overall, while you can find monounsaturated fats in both plant-based foods and animal-based foods. However, plant-based foods are a much better source without a large amount of saturated fat found in animal-based ingredients. In fact, some studies have found that the plant-based sources of monounsaturated fats may be overall more desirable and effective than the animal-based alternative. The following ingredients are all high in monounsaturated fats, from the order of most intensity to least intensity:

- Olive oil
- Almonds
- Cashews
- Peanuts
- Pistachios
- Olives
- Pumpkin Seeds
- Pork
- Avocados
- Sunflower Seeds
- Eggs

As you can see from reading on the various types of fats, the importance of the Mediterranean diet is not only on the food groups you eat but the quality of the ingredients themselves. The fats within meats, cheese, and eggs are overall of lesser quality. Sure, these ingredients may contain a small number of monounsaturated fats, but overall this is overpowered by the sheer number of saturated fats that they contain.

The quality of ingredients does not solely apply to fats and the products that contain these fats, either. Along with the type of fat you consume, an incredibly powerful and important aspect of the Mediterranean diet is the antioxidants that it contains. A stunning example of the antioxidants contained within the Mediterranean comes from the triad of main components: olive oil, bread, and wine. Wine is especially strong in some important antioxidants, and olives and their oil contain many antioxidants, as well.

But first, to understand why the inclusion of antioxidants in the Mediterranean diet is so important, you need to understand how they affect free radicals and oxidative stress. Free radicals are produced through a process of chemical reactions within our own cells and when we are exposed to toxins. These free radicals can be formed when we are exposed to cigarettes, pollution, radiation, sunlight, and other potential toxins. However, they are also formed by the everyday process of converting the food we have eaten into energy for our cells.

The problem is that these free radicals are incredibly unstable. While our body's natural electrons come in pairs that communicate with one another, free radicals contain a single electron. The electrons within free radicals will then attempt to steal the signals from our body's natural electrons for themselves. This process causes massive cellular damage, known as oxidative stress or damage. Soon, oxidative stress causes the production of more free radicals, which increases damage, and in turn the production of even more free radicals.

As this production of free radicals is a part of everyday life in humans, animals, and even plants, we have defenses against the damage they cause. However, for some of us, the damage may far outweigh our body's natural defense system. When our body is unable to confront all of the free radicals assault it the result is lasting cellular damage and cell death. This process damages our very DNA, which can weaken cellular walls, allowing more harmful toxins and substances to enter the body. Another side effect of this cellular damage if plaque buildup in the arteries, leading to cardiovascular disease and heart attacks. When this cellular damage occurs within the brain it is known to cause Alzheimer's disease and other neurological diseases. Lastly, one of the most well-known side effects of large-scale oxidative damage and the toll it takes on our DNA is the development of cancer.

Thankfully, there is a way we can fight back against the onslaught of free radicals we are assaulted with on a daily basis. There are many types of antioxidants which are able to directly negate the free radicals within our systems. These antioxidants come in many forms, but they all help defend us in one way or another. Antioxidants are able to do this by confronting them in one of three ways: they either render free radicals harmless, cause the breakdown of the free radicals themselves, or they give these free radicals they electrons they are seeking in order to help stabilize them better.

Whichever of these methods the antioxidants utilize, they aid in protecting the body from damage by preventing the disastrous effects brought about by the free radicals and their chain reaction of oxidative stress. Antioxidants are empowered with the ability to detoxify the body from these free radicals, in the process preventing disease and decreasing the speed of aging.

Studies are continuously being conducted to learn exactly how antioxidants are able to prevent oxidative stress, as well as how oxidative stress promotes diseases and aging. For instance, researchers are further learning the links between oxidative stress and diseases such as Alzheimer's, Parkinson's, specific forms of cancer, cardiovascular diseases, and much more. By conducting these studies researchers have come to better understand how the antioxidant-rich Mediterranean diet can help in preventing these diseases, as well as how to further prevent them in the future.

There are many types of antioxidants within foods, such as polyphenols, resveratrol, carotenoids, and glutathione. We are able to get polyphenols from berries, resveratrol from grapes, carotenoids from sweet potatoes and carrots, and glutathione from garlic and avocados. Of course, there are many other sources for these antioxidants, as well. Oftentimes, the fruits and vegetables with the most color contain the largest number of antioxidants.

Because these ingredients and others are regularly included on the Mediterranean diet, people eating this way often consume many more antioxidants than their peers. In 2005, the American Journal of Clinical Nutrition published the ATTICA study. This study compared the antioxidant capacity of individuals in Greece. The researchers soon found that those in Greece who followed the standard Mediterranean diet had an antioxidant capacity eleven percent higher than their peers who were not on the standard Mediterranean diet. The same study also found that those on the standard Mediterranean diet experienced a decreased amount of cholesterol in the blood. Overall, most of those on the Mediterranean diet experienced a nineteen percent lower level of harmful LDL cholesterol and reduced levels of heart disease.

Sadly, taking antioxidants on their own, in supplement form outside of a healthy diet, has shown to be ineffective. Many of these antioxidants are present as phytonutrients, which are plant compounds that are neither vitamins nor minerals. While researchers have been able to isolate many of these phytonutrients, the researchers have found that they often have a synergistic effect with one another. This means that outside of a varied and full diet they are unable to benefit the body in the same way. The variety of phytonutrients and antioxidants that are eaten on the Mediterranean diet are able to benefit our health much more than any supplement.

Chapter 3: The Health Benefits of Going Mediterranean

By increasing healthy fats, antioxidants, and phytonutrients, the Mediterranean diet is able to greatly impact health at the cellular level. Studies have time and time again found that this lifestyle can decrease disease and promote healthy aging. Whether you currently have or hope to prevent yourself from having diabetes, cancer, heart disease, or Alzheimer's, the Mediterranean lifestyle can help. In this chapter, we will go over some of the most prominent diseases and how the Mediterranean diet has been proven to help prevent them from occurring. However, we will also explore how people who already have these conditions may utilize the Mediterranean diet in order to treat their symptoms and manage their diseases. You don't have to simply accept that you have one of the most common diseases in the Western world. With the Mediterranean diet, you can change your health for the better and improve your life.

Diabetes

Affecting Over Thirty-Million Americans and the Seventh Leading Cause of Death

The Mediterranean diet has been studied extensively for the treatment of diabetes. During one of these studies, published in the American Journal of Clinical Nutrition in 2013, the Mediterranean diet was compared to other diets frequently recommended for the treatment of this dangerous disease. This study, which was conducted in the United Kingdom, compared vegan, vegetarian, high-protein, low-carbohydrate, high-fiber, low-glycemic index diet, and the Mediterranean diet. Overwhelmingly the Mediterranean diet came out as the most successful in the treatment of diabetes.

During this study, it was found that those on the low-carbohydrate, low-glycemic, high-protein, and Mediterranean diets all experienced improved blood sugar management. These individuals experienced lower A1C scores, which means that over a period of three months their blood sugar averaged at a lower level.

However, the study found that the individuals on the Mediterranean diet experienced great improvements. These people were able to better improve their cholesterol, insulin sensitivity, weight loss, and cardiovascular health.

Another study, published in August of 2009, found that the Mediterranean diet improves the symptoms and management of type II diabetes more than a low-fat diet. This study found that the Mediterranean diet may help individuals to control their type II diabetes without the use of medication, under the control of a knowledgeable physician.

One of the most extensive studies on the Mediterranean diet and type II diabetes as of yet was conducted in Italy. In this study, it was found that the group of individuals who consumed a Mediterranean diet full of whole grains; vegetables; and a minimum of thirty percent of their calories from fats, which mostly comprised of olive oil; were able to significantly increase the management of their disease without the use of medication. This group was compared against a group of individuals on a low-fat diet who consumed no more than thirty percent of their calories from sources of fat. Of these fats, less than ten percent originated from saturated fats.

The study continued for four years, after which it was found that while seventy percent of those on the low-fat diet required medication to control their blood sugar, only forty-four percent of the group on the Mediterranean diet required blood sugar medication.

This study is one of the longest running of its kind, proving the effectiveness of the Mediterranean diet for those with diabetes and pre-diabetes. The study contained two-hundred and fifteen individuals with type II diabetes who were recently diagnosed, overweight, and had never been treated with blood sugar medication. All of these individuals were randomly assigned to a different group, either the low-fat diet group or the Mediterranean diet group.

On the low-fat diet, the participants followed the guidelines established by the American Association. The diet included a large number of whole grains, and greatly limited sweets and fats. The daily fat consumption consisted of no more than thirty- percent of their caloric intake. Of the fat consumed, no more than ten percent originated from saturated fats, such as those occurring in animal-based ingredients.

The individuals on the Mediterranean diet consumed a rich variety of whole grains and vegetables while replacing a large portion of their red meat consumption with both fish and poultry. Overall, this group's diet consisted of a minimum of thirty percent calories originating from fat and no more than fifty percent of their calories originating from carbohydrates.

Some of the proven health benefits for those with type II diabetes on the Mediterranean diet include:

- Lowered blood pressure
- Improved control of blood glucose/sugar levels
- Lower blood cholesterol
- Reduced risk of cardiovascular disease and heart-related deaths
- Healthier blood-lipid profile

- Lower blood triglycerides

- Higher HDL/good cholesterol

- Reduced sugar highs and lows

- Lower risk of developing microvascular disorders in the eyes

- Increased weight loss

Overall, there are many benefits to going on the Mediterranean diet for your health, especially if you have diabetes or are at high risk of developing it in the future. Many people have found benefit with this lifestyle, especially as it is one of the easiest plans to stick to.

Cardiovascular Disease

Affecting Eighty-Four Million Americans and the Leading Cause of Death in Both Men and Women

It is well-known that eating whole-grains and cereals, fatty fish such as salmon and sardines, and only a small amount of low-fat dairy and meat is good for heart health. People with heart conditions often receive advice such as this. However, while we know that a diet rich in heart-healthy ingredients is good for you, there is more to it than simply adding a few ingredients into your preexisting diet.

If you continue to eat a diet that is high in sodium and saturated fats, and you simply add in some more olive oil, salmon, and brown rice, then your heart health and overall health is unlikely to improve as much as it could. Changing your heart health is about more than merely adding in a few ingredients. Rather, you need to make a lifestyle change for the better. This means that you need to comprehensively change your eating pattern, exercise routine, improve your sleep quality, and ensure you stay properly hydrated.

However, on the Mediterranean diet, you are not carelessly adding olive oil and fish to your diet while allowing the remainder to linger unchanged. Instead, you focus on overall changing the way in which you eat, choosing foods that are not only better for your heart and overall health, but that taste good, as well. I don't know about you, but I rarely hear someone complain about pasta tossed with marinara, garlic, olive oil, and seafood or chicken. These days most people can't get enough of hummus. You can always enjoy a salad bursting with avocado, olives, and chicken, as well. To sum it up, there is no lack of flavor or options on the Mediterranean diet. We mentioned earlier that the Mediterranean diet was found to be the easiest diet to stick to. This is especially important for people who have lived their entire lives on a standard Western diet and are unsure how to eat in any other way. The simplicity of the Mediterranean diet will enable anybody, young or old, to attain better heart health.

While we know that some of the ingredients that compose the Mediterranean diet are good for heart health, how does this diet comprehensively improve heart health for the better? This has been a question in the scientific and health communities for many years. Some researchers have even described the Mediterranean diet as a black box, as researchers have known the evidence proving its effectiveness, but have not understood why it is so effective.

Thankfully, with the completion of more studies, scientists have compiled more evidence and have begun to understand more of the reasoning behind the effectiveness of this lifestyle.

One of the most comprehensive studies on heart disease and the Mediterranean diet was published in December of 2018. This study assessed the risk factors and biomarkers which are associated with heart disease in women consuming the Mediterranean diet. This study utilized blood samples and questionnaires in order to study over twenty-five thousand women long-term. In fact, this study is so comprehensive that it took place over a period of twelve years.

The participants of the study were categorized based on their observance to the Mediterranean diet as either low, middle, or high observance. Over the course of the twelve-year study, researchers observed four-hundred and twenty-eight women in the low group, three-hundred and fifty-six in the middle group, and two-hundred and forty-six in the high group. By observing various groups, the researchers were able to find that the middle group experienced a twenty-three percent reduction in cardiovascular disease risk than the low group, and the high group experienced a twenty-eight percent reduction.

After analyzing biomarkers for glucose metabolism, insulin resistance, inflammation, and heart disease at both the beginning and the end of the study, the researchers were able to get a clearer picture of how the Mediterranean diet affects heart disease. The researchers found that the women who followed the Mediterranean diet the closest experienced an average twenty-five percent decrease in heart disease, compared to the women who followed the lifestyle less rigorously.

These results helped researchers to understand that the Mediterranean diet is able to greatly aid in the treatment of heart disease by targeting chronic inflammation. This is important as inflammation is one of the biggest risk factors contributing to the cause and worsening of heart disease. It was also found that the Mediterranean diet can contribute to improved heart health by lessening body fat and improving both insulin resistance and glucose metabolism.

This study further strengthens the results of previous studies, in which researchers studied the blood biomarkers of people on the Mediterranean diet. In these studies, people were similarly separated into low, middle, and high groups according to how strictly they followed the diet. The biggest biomarker change was inflammation, which reduced by twenty-nine percent. Similarly, body mass index, insulin resistance, and glucose metabolism all experienced a twenty-seven percent reduced risk.

In 2013, a study on the benefits of the Mediterranean diet was published. This study compared the differences of a low-fat diet (which didn't allow high-fat ingredients such as oil, nuts, or fatty meats) to two types of Mediterranean diets: the first type included the addition of thirty grams of mixed nuts daily. The second type included the addition of a minimum of four tablespoons of extra virgin olive oil daily. Participants in this study included seven-thousand four-hundred and forty-seven individuals, all of whom were at high risk of heart disease but currently free of the conditions. At the beginning of the study, the participants were between the ages of fifty-five and eighty and maintained their assigned diets for five years.

Sadly, this study came under question for a time. The researchers ended up withdrawing their findings as they incorrectly carried out the study. The biggest error that the researchers made was in not randomly assigning all of the participants to the diets, which could have possibly affected the results.

Thankfully, these results were re-analyzed by researchers, while taking the error into consideration. After analyzing the data again these researchers found that the results were similar and that the Mediterranean diet with either the addition of extra virgin olive oil and mixed nuts reduces the risk of heart events by an average thirty percent. Overall, the Mediterranean diet greatly decreases stroke, heart attacks, and heart-related deaths compared to a low-fat diet.

Large clinical and observational studies have also observed other aspects of how the Mediterranean diet affects heart health, along with other common diseases such as cancer. These studies highlight the importance of the Mediterranean diet in a world that is overrun with heart disease. While many people realize that heart disease and heart attacks are dangerous, overall many people are unaware of just how deadly and common these conditions are. Heart attacks affect seven-hundred thirty-five thousand Americans annually. Six-hundred and ten-thousand Americans die of heart disease annually. While men are usually the center of conversation when it comes to heart disease, they are almost nearly as common in women. Because of this, heart disease is a leading cause of death in both men and women.

It's easy to brush off a problem and tell yourself that you'll take care of your heart health "later." It's simple to not worry about it until after you've had a heart attack if you survive. Don't put off until tomorrow what may save your life. Really pay attention to these words and the scientific evidence.

Large cohort studies on the Mediterranean diet have shown that through strictly adhering to the lifestyle a person can greatly reduce their vascular inflammation markers and blood pressure levels. As we have explained, there is no one factor of the Mediterranean diet that promotes these health benefits. You can't simply pour olive oil on all of your meals and hope to improve your heart health. However, the benefits of olive oil remain, and when paired with a full Mediterranean diet can be quite astounding. This is primarily because extra virgin olive oil is not only a monounsaturated fat, but it contains many of the beneficial elements of the fruit it is derived from. Some of these elements include lipophilic compounds, phenolic compounds, and α-tocopherol. These components have strong anti-inflammatory and antioxidant properties, which will directly impact your heart health.

Cancer

One Million, Seven Hundred Thirty-Five Thousand and Three Hundred Fifty Americans in 2018 Alone

If that statistic isn't scary, I don't know what is. Worldwide cancer is affecting millions of people. While more people are able to survive with increasing medical care, much of this care is incredibly painful and difficult to go through. We need to continue to search for a cure for cancer, but we should also find ways in which to prevent this devastating disease. One way in which we can lower our risk of developing cancer is with the Mediterranean diet. This isn't surprising, as free radicals and oxidative stress cause the formation of cancer cells, and the Mediterranean diet combats this directly by increasing the number of antioxidants within our bodies.

Cancer cells are able to thrive in the human body for multiple reasons, but one of these reasons is due to their ability to escape death. While most cells eventually die and are replaced with healthy cells, cancer cells inhibit this process so that they can continue to grow and spread. However, this ability of these deadly cells may be stopped. Researchers have found that by including specific plant-based foods we can alter our gene regulation, which transforms the cancer cells from super-powered cells able to take over into cells that can simply die as they naturally should.

The compound that can alter cancer cells to such a degree is known as apigenin and is found in a variety of fruits, vegetables, and herbs. This compound is especially known to be present in parsley, chamomile, celery, spinach, artichokes, licorice root, peppermint, and red wine.

Researchers are still left to puzzle out how many ingredients benefit the human body, even if their benefits have already been proven. It can be difficult to find the exact cause as what molecules and systems in the human body these compounds affect. Still, scientists have found that apigenin is able to bind to approximately one-hundred and sixty proteins within the body. This suggests that similar nutrients may have other helpful benefits that we are not yet aware of. This could be powerful since most pharmaceutical medications only target a single molecule rather than dozens or even hundreds.

While we all know that we need to eat healthily, it is much easier to do so when we have a specific reason and know how and why it is helping. This is partially why knowing about apigenin and how it affects cancer cells is beneficial. It can also help to have this knowledge so that you can ensure you are eating a large number of foods containing this compound.

A study published in JAMA Internal Medicine found that women who eat a traditional Mediterranean diet with the addition of extra virgin olive oil are less likely to develop breast cancer. This study was run in conjunction with another one, both of which were conducted in Spain, which found that people who eat a Mediterranean diet are thirty percent less likely to develop strokes, heart attacks, or to die from heart-related causes. The researchers tracked about four-thousand three hundred women between the ages of sixty and eighty. During this time, they noted which women developed breast cancer so that they could know if it correlated depending on the group they were in. There were three diet groups the women were divided between—the low-fat, the Mediterranean with extra olive oil, and the Mediterranean with added nuts.

Of the women in the study thirty-five were diagnosed with breast cancer through the course of the trial. The women in the Mediterranean diet group with extra virgin olive oil added experienced a sixty-two percent decrease in cancer than the women on the low-fat diet. The women with the nut addition experienced little statistical difference from the low-fat group, which shows the importance olive oil plays in the Mediterranean diet.

Larger studies of this kind need to be conducted, as this study was only able to analyze thirty-five women with breast cancer, but the results are exciting.

A study conducted over a twenty-year period in the Netherlands on sixty-thousand menopausal women between the ages of fifty-five to sixty-nine found positive results. This study found that by eating a Mediterranean diet postmenopausal women can reduce their risk of developing breast cancer by forty percent.

The researchers collected data on over two-thousand women who developed breast cancer and then compared them against women with similar lifestyle and diet practices who did not develop this type of cancer. Not surprisingly, the researchers found that there is no evidence that the Mediterranean diet may increase breast cancer. In fact, their findings were quite the opposite as they found that the diet can greatly reduce the risk of breast cancer. However, the findings did reveal that the Mediterranean diet is especially powerful in reducing the risk of developing a specific type of breast cancer, known as estrogen receptor-positive breast cancer.

While most of the studies on the Mediterranean diet and cancer are specifically targeting breast cancer, that doesn't mean that the Mediterranean diet can't prevent other forms of cancer as well. In fact, one study found that this lifestyle can reduce the risk of developing colorectal cancer.

For the purpose of this study researchers examined over eight-hundred individuals who were having either colonoscopies or screenings completed. The participants ranged between forty and seventy years of age under an average risk of developing colorectal cancer. Their lifestyle factors, diet, height, and body mass index were all assessed. Polyps are abnormal growths on mucus membrane, this is what can potentially lead to colorectal cancer. The American Cancer Society refers to some of these polyps as having "high-grade dysplasia," which means that they look abnormal are resemble cancerous polyps.

The researchers studied control subjects who had never had polyps against those with high-grade dysplasia polyps. By comparing the various risk factors, the researchers were soon able to find that those with the worst polyps adopted fewer of the Mediterranean diet's components. By adopting as few as two or three Mediterranean diet components individuals were able to reduce their risk of high-grade dysplasia polyps by a significant fifty percent. This reduction in developing colorectal cancer is further reduced by adopting more of the Mediterranean diet's components.

The components of the Mediterranean diet which researchers found made the most impact on colorectal cancer and polyps are increased fish and fruit consumption along with decreased soft drink consumption. Each of these three components was associated with an average thirty percent reduced risk. People who met all three of these criteria reduced their risk of developing colorectal cancer by nearly eighty-six percent.

Lastly, there was a meta-analysis published in late 2017, which evaluated the risks of developing specific cancers, their mortality rates, and risk of cancer recurrence when on the Mediterranean diet. This meta-analyses evaluated eighty-three studies and overall over two million participants.

The results of the meta-analyses showed universally lower rates of cancer mortality with those who attained a stricter Mediterranean diet. This included studies on breast, colorectal, gastric, liver, head and neck, and prostate cancers. After analyzing the various components of the Mediterranean diet it was found that an increase in plant-based foods (namely grains, fruits, and vegetables) were most to thank for the decreased risk.

There are many reasons to go on the Mediterranean diet. Whether you hope to lose weight, lower your blood pressure, improve the aging of your brain, or decrease your risk of developing either cancer, heart disease, or diabetes, the Mediterranean diet may help. It may take a lifestyle adjustment, but it has been shown that the Mediterranean diet is the easiest to stick to with some of the most powerful benefits, as well.

Now that you have a fundamental understanding of the reasons why you should choose the Mediterranean diet, in the remainder of this book, we will examine how best to undertake your new lifestyle change.

Chapter 4: Using the Mediterranean Diet for Effective Weight Loss

People try diet after diet in search of a plan where they can lose weight. They hop from Weight Watchers to Atkins, from the South Beach Diet to SlimFast. They may even try the Master Cleanse where they eat nothing—choosing to instead drink saltwater, lemonade, and a laxative herbal tea. While on these diets, many people lose weight. They boast of losing five, ten, fifteen, or maybe even thirty pounds. The problem is that these pounds make their way back—often sooner rather than later.

However, that is not the only problem. In exchange for yo-yo dieting, people become malnourished and wreck their metabolisms. This causes a person with a likely already slow metabolism to only slow it further, turning it from a slow walk to a turtle's pace, and it may eventually reach a snail's pace. For this reason, many people will lose a small amount of weight while on the newest diet trend but continue to pack on the pounds over the years. For all their years of dieting all they have to show is a steadily increasing waistline and number on the scale.

Losing weight doesn't have to be this way. You can gain both health and a slimmer figure. Whether your goal in coming to the Mediterranean diet was to get more fit, treat or prevent disease, or reach your desired pant size, you will find that this lifestyle has the answers you are looking for.

It's important to know that losing your weight and gaining health doesn't have to be mutually exclusive. Due to the surge of fad and crash diets which cause people to drop weight quickly while also losing health it may seem as if the two can't coincide.

However, any diet that promotes long-term weight loss and is maintainable will also focus on health. The Mediterranean diet does just this very thing.

You can believe that the Mediterranean diet is maintainable. Not only has the World Health Organization ranked it as the most maintainable diet, but it's a complete lifestyle that has been used for centuries. People throughout countries in the Mediterranean have used this way of eating every day of their lives prior to the 1960s when the amount of junk food and fast food increased worldwide. Just as the people in the Mediterranean were able to live this way, and many still do, people in modern times and throughout the world can also maintain this lifestyle.

Although, you don't have to just believe me, as there's plenty of science that backs up the weight loss potential and maintainability of the Mediterranean diet. For example, The American Journal of Medicine published a study on this very subject in 2016. This study found that on the Mediterranean diet people are able to lose an average of nine to twenty-two pounds and maintain their weight loss for at least a year.

Another two-year study analyzed over three-hundred obese men at an average of fifty-two years old. This study placed the men on various diets, including a low-fat and non-restricted calorie diet, a low-carbohydrate and restricted calorie diet, and lastly the Mediterranean diet with restricted calories.

In this study the low-fat group lost an average of just over six pounds, the low-carbohydrate group lost just over ten pounds, and the Mediterranean group lost just over nine and a half pounds each. Of the people in the study thirty-six were diagnosed with diabetes. The participants with diabetes who were placed on the Mediterranean diet experienced the most improvement in diabetes symptoms and levels. While both the Mediterranean diet and the low-carbohydrate diet had comparable weight loss results, overall the Mediterranean diet has been proven to be the most maintainable. For this reason, a person is more likely to keep the weight off with the Mediterranean diet rather than with the low-carbohydrate diet.

A meta-analysis comparing the results of sixteen controlled and randomized studies analyzed the results of nearly three-thousand and five hundred participants. In these studies, individuals were placed in groups both on the Mediterranean diet and on control diets. The results found that people on the Mediterranean diet regularly experienced weight loss when compared to other diets. This lifestyle was found to be most effective when continued for longer than six months, when paired with healthy physical activity, and when calories are watched in order to prevent overeating. Studies have long shown the vegetarians and vegans who focus on healthy whole foods such as grains, legumes, nuts, seeds, fruits, vegetables, and healthy fats are on average must healthier than the general population and at a lower risk of being obese or overweight. While the Mediterranean diet is definitely not vegan or vegetarian, it is a largely plant-based diet where you focus more on foods that were grown than those originating from animals. Yes, you can still eat fish, seafood, chicken, eggs, and a dairy, but many of these ingredients you will eat in moderation due to their saturated fats. Due to prioritizing plant-based foods the Mediterranean diet has been proven to regularly produce greater weight loss results than the low-fat and many other diets. Not only that, but the weight loss achieved on the Mediterranean diet specifically can aid in the loss of stubborn belly fat. You will find this is incredibly important as belly fat is the most dangerous type of fat, which can lead to metabolic syndrome, heart disease, and type II diabetes.

However, it's important to not replace your usual number of animal-based ingredients with refined carbohydrates. Remember, the focus is on healthy whole ingredients, not refined flours and sugars. Similarly, just because honey is allowed on the Mediterranean diet doesn't mean you can eat it regularly. Prior to the 1960s honey was a special treat in the Mediterranean diet, not an everyday occurrence. Instead, if the people wanted something sweet they would often enjoy fruit for dessert. This doesn't mean you can't enjoy honey, but try to limit it to a couple of times a week.

While you can certainly enjoy plenty of fish and seafood, and a moderate amount of chicken and low-fat dairy, on the Mediterranean diet, try to not replace all of your regular protein sources with these ingredients. Instead, focus on plant-based proteins such as legumes and whole-grains. This is the way in which the standard Mediterranean diet was eaten and part of what makes it such a success. This is not merely speculation but has been proven in studies.

A 2015 study on over one-hundred thousand individuals study found that for each extra daily serving of fruit people lost about half a pound of weight. The same study also found that for each serving of non-starchy vegetables participants were able to lose a quarter-pound of fat.

Researchers found that part of the cause for this is that when you increase your high-fiber vegetable intake you will feel more full and therefore eat fewer high-calorie foods. You will also feel more full from consuming healthy monounsaturated fats, such as those found in olive oil, leading you to be full and fully nourished while naturally consuming fewer calories than you otherwise would.

However, while the Mediterranean diet is highly successful for weight loss, in order to get the most out of the diet and its weight loss benefits there are some things you need to keep in mind. Just as you don't want to go overboard on the amount of honey you are eating, there are other lifestyle factors, tips, and tricks that you should keep in mind. Don't worry, these are not difficult, but they are impactful. By making a few changes to your daily life you can drastically improve your weight loss, reduce your mental stress, increase your health, and improve upon the ease of the Mediterranean diet. Following you will find different ways in which you can improve your Mediterranean diet and overall life, health, wellness, and weight.

Create a Lifestyle Change, Not a Diet Change

The term "Mediterranean diet" may have the word "diet" in it, but it is more of an overall lifestyle rather than a diet. For this reason, you want to make changes to many areas of your life, more than simply what you eat or how much you eat.

Most fad and crash diets are completed by the very same people. For instance, if a person has tried Weight Watchers they have also likely tried other popular diets such as Paleo, the Ketogenic diet, the South Beach diet, and the Master Cleanse. This is because many people get into the habit of yo-yo dieting, where they try one diet for a time, "give up," and then try another. It is not their fault for "giving up" on these diets, because these diets are unmaintainable. These diets usually con people into believing that they can lose a lot of weight quickly. However, after a person is on these diets for a time, their weight loss stalls or they are simply unable to maintain the strict and unhealthy eating style.

Instead of believing you will do the Mediterranean diet for a short time, lose a lot of weight, and then go back to a standard Western diet, go into this lifestyle for the long haul. If you want the weight loss and health benefits of the Mediterranean lifestyle, then you must stick with it.

However, don't worry. Unlike the crash and fad diets, we have mentioned the Mediterranean lifestyle is maintainable. You can enjoy a rich and varied diet while completely satisfied with your meals and the flavors they contain. After all, who doesn't enjoy a diet that includes pasta, avocados, and wine?

In order to make these lifestyle changes, you want to set realistic goals that are attainable. People will often set goals such as "lose twenty pounds in a month." The problem is that this weight loss pace is only possible when on a crash diet or when extremely ill. While crash diets claim to help you lose fifteen, twenty, or more calories a month, you will find that by losing weight this quickly it is unmaintainable and before long you will gain that weight, and then some, back.

It's also important to keep in mind that such rapid weight loss is unhealthy. Your liver is unable to healthfully handle rapid weight loss, and it can become incredibly detrimental for your health. Lastly, if you lose weight too quickly you will find that you get sagging skin, which doesn't give you the slim figure you are hoping for. Instead, doctors recommend losing between two to three pounds a week, which averages out to eight to twelve pounds a month.

If you are one of the many people living a fast-paced lifestyle, then you will have to focus on making time in your schedule to eat well. When we are busy it is all too easy to grab fast food on the way home or while running errands. If we had a stressful day we might pull ice cream out of the freezer rather than eating a healthy snack. On the way to work, we might grab a doughnut and coffee rather than taking the time to prepare breakfast.

I get it. Life is busy and most people are always on the run. However, if we want to live a healthy life and lose weight, we have to make time for what is important. You are important, your health is important, and your weight loss goals are important. Make time for yourself instead of sacrificing yourself for your schedule.

Now, this doesn't mean you can't continue advancing at work, taking time for school, or caring for your kids. You simply need to find a time you can set aside to prepare some meals and get a little bit of exercise in. This doesn't have to be time-consuming, there are many ways in which you can easily prepare ingredients for use, later on, to assemble quick meals on the go. You can even make yourself Mediterranean lunch boxes to keep with you to eat wherever the road might take you.

Later on in this book, you will be provided with a two-week meal plan. This meal plan will include many easy and quick to assemble meals and snacks. Use this meal plan to help you figure out how to better set aside time for yourself and your goal of improved health and weight.

When beginning the Mediterranean diet, you don't have to jump in all at once. While some people may prefer this method, to others it can become overwhelming. Therefore, look at your life and find small changes you can make to slowly guide yourself into a more Mediterranean lifestyle.

For instance, if you always drink a sugary or diet soda in the afternoons you can try giving that up first. If you always keep ice cream in the freezer or cookies in the pantry to stop buying them.

Maybe you are a person who loves red meat, try slowly replacing it with fish, seafood, and chicken.

If you drink alcohol try switching the type you drink to red wine. While most types of alcohol don't provide health benefits, there is a wealth of benefits to drinking a glass of red wine a day.

If you are someone who never gives a thought to exercise, try to add a workout or two to your week. You can start slow by simply walking around the block, walking in your home with a workout DVD, or attempting a light workout at the gym. It doesn't matter if you only start out walking a single mile or for ten minutes. By starting slowly your body will have time to adjust and before long you will find that you can gradually increase the pace and intensity.

Overall, you want to create small changes in your life that you can maintain and that will stick. If you jump in head first you may get mixed up and not know what side is up or down. However, if you slowly wade into the pool of the Mediterranean diet you will find that you can keep your head above the water and before long you will be swimming naturally. Go at your own pace, slowly adding in more Mediterranean aspects to your lifestyle.

Adjust the Way You Think About Calories

Oftentimes, people who have a past of yo-yo dieting have been taught to obsess over calories. They try to consume as few calories as possible while dieting and are always checking the labels of their ingredients. This will often lead to people choosing low-calorie "diet" food rather than healthy choices such as avocados, olive oil, and sardines.

However, calories are important. Our cells require the energy from these calories in order to function at the most basic of levels. Not only do we need these calories for running, walking, cooking, working, and exercising, we also need them for our most basic functions such as breathing and to keep our heart beating.

Everyone has a different metabolic rate, which is how quickly they burn through calories. This is the reason why some people may consume twelve-hundred calories a day while others require twenty-two hundred. This metabolic rate depends upon your age, height, weight, gender, activity level, genetics, and overall health.

If you hope to lose weight, then you need to ensure that your calorie consumption meets your needs rather than exceeding them. If you require eighteen-hundred calories to maintain weight, then twenty-two hundred would cause you to gain weight. This is because excess calories are stored as fat for use later on.

However, this doesn't mean you need to obsess over calories as you have been taught on fad and crash diets. By making simple lifestyle changes you will find that your calorie count can naturally level out to your body's requirements. You can do this by focusing on eating more high-fiber vegetables, replacing excess meat with whole grains and legumes, exercising regularly, and not mindlessly snacking. You will find that by doing this you are more satisfied and full, leading you to naturally eat what your body requires and unlikely more.

Although, if you find that your weight loss stalls for a number of weeks you may want to pay more attention to your calories. You can find many calculators online to determine how many calories you should eat to either lose, maintain, or gain weight. Use one of these calculators to get a general idea of where you should be at, and then pay attention to what you eat. You might find that you are eating more fruits than vegetables. Maybe you're adding creamer to your coffee, which is not only adding up calorie wise but is also adding saturated fats to your diet.

Perhaps you are mindlessly adding olive oil and avocados to many of your dishes. While these two ingredients are certainly healthy, filling, and part of the Mediterranean diet, you have to be careful. Remember, high-fat ingredients such as olives, olive oil, avocados, and nuts are also high in calories. If we add more of these to our diets than we realize the weight can quickly stall. Therefore, notice how much you are eating so that you can be more aware of what your body requires.

Prioritize Exercise

Research has shown that diet alone won't help in weight loss. In fact, people who double up on exercise without controlling their diet are likely to overeat due to the body signaling that it needs to refuel after working out. Instead, it's important to pair manageable exercise with a healthy diet. In fact, part of the basis of the Mediterranean diet includes a moderate activity. This is because prior to the 1960s people in the Mediterranean, specifically, the island of Crete in Greece would live active lifestyles in order to walk to their destinations, to cook, clean, and work in the fields. This exercise not only increases the burning of calories, but it promotes overall good health and can aid in healing a damaged metabolism.

In a study on over five-hundred thousand people, it was found that eating a Mediterranean diet can decrease your chance of dying early by twenty percent. Another study found that by completing thirty minutes of moderate exercise most days of the week you can reduce your risk of early death by twenty-five percent. The people in this study who practiced vigorous exercise for twenty minutes three times a week were able to reduce their risk of death by thirty-three percent.

Yet another study found that with the Mediterranean diet and regular exercise people who smoke or are overweight can still benefit overall, even if they don't give up smoking or lose weight. This proves that by combining the Mediterranean diet and exercise into a lifestyle you can reduce your overall risk of early death, including those caused by heart disease. This study was quite conclusive, as it was conducted with the help of over five-hundred and sixty-six thousand, and four-hundred participants. All of the participants were between the ages of fifty and seventy-one.

Both the women and men within this study experienced a decrease in deaths. Overall the risk of men dying of cancer reduced by seventeen percent and the risk of cardiovascular-related deaths reduced by twenty-two percent. For women, the risk of dying from cancer reduced fourteen percent while the risk of cardiovascular-related death reduced by twenty-one percent.

The same study tracked people's death rates compared to their activity levels. The participants who practiced thirty minutes of moderate exercise most days of the week were twenty-seven percent less likely to die young than those who didn't exercise. Similarly, those who practiced twenty minutes of vigorous exercise three times a week were thirty-two percent less likely to die young. A smaller amount of weekly activity still helped in reducing death risks, it was shown to reduce the risk of early death by nineteen percent.

Another study found that people who eat a Mediterranean diet, live an active lifestyle, and watch their calories are able to lose weight and maintain the weight loss after a year of beginning the diet. This shows that the Mediterranean diet, when paired with exercise, is not only effective in weight loss but effective in keeping the weight off down the road.

However, how do you include physical activity into your life? You can certainly practice bodybuilding, CrossFit, or HIIT programs. While vigorous exercise a couple of times a week can improve your health, if you are unable to complete vigorous activities, that's okay. There are many moderate exercises which you can include within your daily life, boosting your weight loss and improving your health in the process.

Two of the best options for those who are tight on time or energy is cardio and flexibility routines. With these options, you can find many different workout methods that you can do at home, around the block, in the neighborhood park, at the gym, or in a class. If one of these exercises doesn't fit your needs, you can always switch things up and find another option that will help aid your body and weight loss in a similar manner. For instance, if you want to do cardio but struggle with a stair climber then you might try swimming or cycling instead.

Whether you are exercising to lose weight or gain better health and longevity, there are many options for you to choose from. The human body is conditioned to move, yet in our modern society few people have the opportunity to get up and use the muscles, tendons, and other functions they have been given. Instead, many of us sit at a desk all day or stand in the same position. Therefore, it's important to set aside a given time where we can move our bodies in the way that they were created. This doesn't have to be anything strenuous or serious, but it does need to get our body moving for twenty to forty minutes. We can control how we age to a large extent through diet and exercise. Do you want to age in a way that you are sick and stuck in bed or where you are still moving around and capable? The choice is yours.

Whether you choose to complete cardio, flexibility exercises, or both, you can experience many benefits. For instance, cardio has been shown to lessen the risk of strokes by increasing blood flow to the brain. This can also improve memory and increase endorphins, dopamine, serotonin, and norepinephrine. You may also experience improved lung function, increased blood sugar control, improved sleep, increased joint mobility and lessened pain for those with arthritis, healthier skin, and stronger muscles. If you practice regular flexibility exercises you can experience increased muscle strength and tone, a decrease of stress on the joints, increased lung function, improved posture, better sleep, relaxed muscles, improved mental health, reduced stress, and lower chronic inflammation.

Some people may discount flexibility exercises, thinking it's all yoga and Pilates that housewives do in their off time. However, there are many benefits to practicing these exercises young or old, active or non-active. Exercises such as yoga, Pilates, and tai chi have the ability to strengthen the body. Not only that, but if you are someone who worries about aging, practice vigorous exercise, or who competes in sports you will find that these exercises prepare you for the future. By increasing your flexibility, you will be less likely to develop injuries or arthritis as you age. You will be less likely to injure yourself while you are competing in sports or practicing more vigorous exercises. However, with flexibility exercises, like any type of activity, it is best to begin slowly. If you jump right into doing a difficult yoga, Pilates, or tai chi pose then you will injure yourself. Remember, these injuries are not something to be taken lightly. If you tear a tendon it will most likely heal, but you could experience pain from it for your entire life. Therefore, it's important to start with beginner level activities and work your way up.

You can certainly complete these on your own, but if you aren't confident you can always take a class to help you work your way up.

There are many types of cardio exercises you can practice, some of which can even be quite fun! However, it's important to keep in mind that you want to maintain a specific activity level which stimulates your heart and increased blood flow. There is a recommended heart rate for people depending upon their age. To calculate your specific cardio heart range simply remove fifty to seventy percent from the number two-hundred and twenty and then remove your age. This means that if you are thirty-five your target range is seventy-five to one-hundred and nineteen. If you are fifty your target range is sixty to one-hundred and four.

When beginning cardio you can work up to your higher number. For instance, in the beginning, you can target your low number, either seventy-five or sixty with the examples given above. You can start out by hitting this target range for five minutes at a time until you are able to manage this heart rate for an entire twenty to thirty minutes. Afterward, you can gradually begin pushing yourself to increase your heart rate, possibly by five or ten beats a minute. This means that if you have been practicing at seventy-five you can bump it up to eighty or eighty-five.

Some examples of cardio workouts you can practice include the elliptical, climbing stairs or a stair climber device, running, sprinting, cycling, swimming, rowing, kettlebells, jump rope, skating, jumping jacks, burpees, dancing, hiking, boxing, and sports. There is a large number of options when it comes to cardio. You are sure to find one that fits with your interests and lifestyle.

Whatever your motive for losing weight, if you stick to the Mediterranean diet and live an active lifestyle you are sure to find progress. It may not have the same speedy weight loss as a crash diet, but unlike those diets, the weight loss attained on the Mediterranean diet has been proven to be maintainable and long-lasting.

Chapter 5:

The Mediterranean Food Pyramid

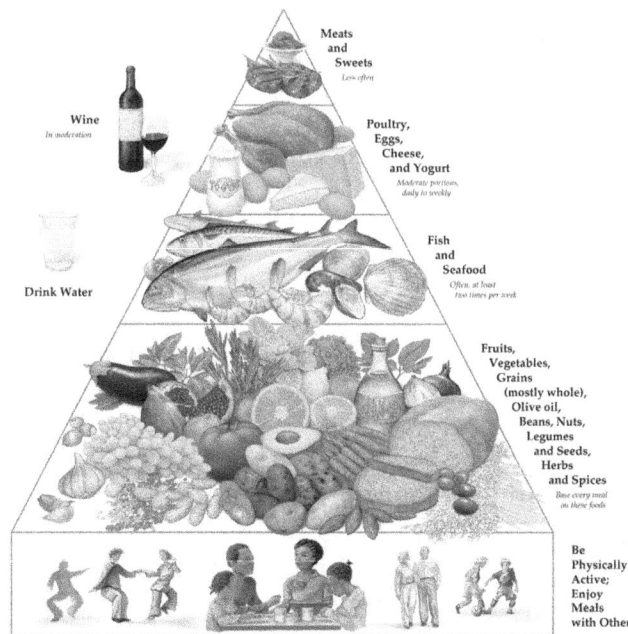

When beginning a new diet or lifestyle, it's helpful to know the science behind it, relevant tips and tricks, and how to increase weight loss. However, one of the most important things for you to know fundamentally is what you should and shouldn't eat. Not only that, but you need to know how much you can eat of specific foods. Obviously, you wouldn't eat sweets as much as you eat vegetables, but what about the grayer areas? Do you eat poultry as much as you eat fish? In this chapter, we will be going over the

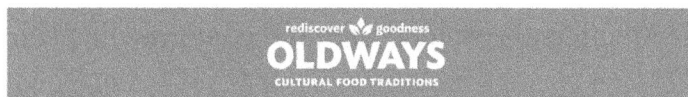

Mediterranean food pyramid from bottom to top. You will learn exactly what is included on the Mediterranean diet, what isn't, and how you should prioritize your pantry. After having a broad overview of the Mediterranean food pyramid, we will go into more detail on specific ingredients, how they should be included, and why.

This is the most used Mediterranean food pyramid, provided by Old Ways and used throughout official government health and wellness recommendations. The first tier on the bottom of the pyramid focuses on living a healthy and active lifestyle where you are getting exercise through work and play. It also recommends enjoying your meals with others, though of course, you can still enjoy a full Mediterranean diet if you are eating alone or with your cat as your only company.

The second tier of the Mediterranean food pyramid contains the primary foods you will be enjoying. This includes vegetables, fruits, grains, beans, legumes, nuts, seeds, herbs, spices, and olive oil. Most of your meals should be comprised primarily of these ingredients.

If you desire you can make Mediterranean-flavored meals, but your pallet is not limited to the flavors from that one cuisine. For instance, you could easily make a Chinese or Mexican dish with these ingredients and have it fit all of the qualifications of the Mediterranean diet. This is because it is about what you are eating rather than the flavors of the food.

Aside from protein originating from grains, legumes, beans, nuts, and seeds, fish and seafood will be your largest source of animal-based protein. This is the third tier of the Mediterranean pyramid. These are important to include on the Mediterranean diet, as they often include many important vitamins, minerals, and other nutrients.

For example, fatty fish such as salmon, sardines, and mackerel contain a large amount of vital omega-6 fatty acids. Most people on the standard Western diet don't get nearly enough of this important fat, which increases chronic inflammation levels. By increasing your omega-6 fat intake you can lower inflammation, in the processing lowering your risk of illnesses such as heart disease, cancer, stroke, diabetes, and more. Try to consume fish and seafood, especially fatty fish, at least two or three times a week.

The fourth tier of the Mediterranean diet pyramid contains poultry, yogurt, cheese, and eggs. These ingredients are only to be eaten in small number, up to a few times a week. You don't want to overdo these ingredients, as they are not as nutritionally beneficial as the lower tier ingredients and they contain saturated fats.

For instance, three ounces of chicken breast contains two grams of saturated fat. A chicken thigh, without the skin, contains two and a half grams. A single egg contains one and a half grams. Lastly, one ounce or slice of sharp cheddar cheese contains five and a half grams! Try to limit these saturated fats and instead promote healthier fats, such as those in olive oil and fatty fish.

The fifth and last tier of the Mediterranean diet contains sweets and non-poultry or fish meat. While you can certainly enjoy some beef or a slice of cake on a rare occasion, it should be a special treat and occur only occasionally, not frequently. Red meat is known to contain a large number of saturated fat and increase the risk of many common diseases, including heart disease. It's important to keep in mind that a three-ounce serving of seventy percent lean ground beef contains nine and a half grams of saturated fat. A single medium-sized steak (two-hundred and fifty grams) contains a whopping twenty-one grams of saturated fat! This is much more than that found within the other animal products allowed on the Mediterranean diet.

While sweets may be enjoyable, they contain no benefits to the human diet and only worsen our immune system, weight, insulin response, immune system, and more. Between the sugar and refined grains, and dairy these ingredients and dishes should be kept to a minimum.

Outside of the Mediterranean diet's pyramid, but of equal importance, is the consumption of water and red wine. Of course, of these two drink options, water is the most important. Many people do not consume enough of this important fluid, becoming dehydrated and increasing the risk of malnutrition. Doctors recommend consuming half of your body's weight in ounces at a minimum. This means that if you weight one-hundred and fifty pounds you will need to drink at the very least seventy-five ounces of water daily. However, don't try to drink most of this water in one sitting to get it over with. Instead, you need to spread out your consumption. The human liver is unable to process more than one liter (four cups) of water within the span of an hour.

Red wine is an important part of a healthy Mediterranean diet and lifestyle. Of course, everyone may not be able to partake. If you have religious misgivings, struggle with alcohol addiction, are underage, take medication counterintuitive with alcohol, or have a health condition negatively affected by its consumption, then you should avoid drinking red wine or any other source of alcohol. Even a small amount of alcohol could negatively affect you if you are struggling with a health condition, taking medication, or have an alcohol addiction.

However, if you are able to partake in alcohol avoid other types and stick with red wine. While other types of alcohol may lead to negative side effects, when drinking in moderation there are many benefits to red wine. Avoid drinking any alcohol, even red wine, excessively. Women should stick with a four-ounce glass and men a four to eight-ounce glass. You can enjoy this red wine daily or weekly.

Now that you have an understanding of the fundamentals of the Mediterranean pyramid let's go tier by tier, discovering the benefits of various components and ingredients that you can enjoy within your daily life. By knowing these ingredients and their benefits you will be able to more easily create simple meals on the go without worry. You will be able to easily mix and match flavors and ingredients for tasty, wholesome, and healthy meals.

The Main Components

While the entire Mediterranean diet is important, the second tier is the one you should use the most. This level of the Mediterranean pyramid contains grains, vegetables, fruits, legumes, beans, nuts, seeds, spices, and olive oil. You will want more of your meals to contain these ingredients. However, it's helpful to know more about these ingredients specifically, so let's have a look at some of the ones you can include in your daily life.

Whole Grains and Cereals

There are many benefits of including whole grains in the Mediterranean diet. You can try grains such as whole wheat, brown rice, bulgur, barley, amaranth, millet, oats, corn, quinoa, rye, spelt, sorghum, kamut, and buckwheat. The benefits of these grains and cereals are numerous. However, at a glance, they add a needed source of vitamins, minerals, fiber, and complex carbohydrates to your diet. That's not even including the flavor and texture boosts they add to dishes, as well as being satisfying while relatively low in calories.

However, the calories in grains and cereals can add up. Therefore, try to eat small servings mixed in with other ingredients such as vegetables and fish. You can easily accomplish this by eating a half cup of whole grains with every meal. You can certainly enjoy pasta on the Mediterranean diet, but try to keep more refined pasta to a minimum. For day-to-day use, you can enjoy whole grain pasta in a variety of dishes and sauces. You may be unfamiliar with cooking grains such as millet, barley, buckwheat, or even quinoa, but don't worry. These grains are easy and quick to cook with a bit of water. You will find that with hardly any time at all cooking these grains becomes natural. Once you learn how to cook these grains you can simply enjoy them on the side of a dish, mix them into sauces, or make a grain and vegetable salad.

You may be wondering why the focus on whole grains and why you can't just stick with regular refined pasta and flours. To understand this, you need a basic understanding of the components that make up various grains.

All grains are made up of three portions when they are in their whole form, these are the bran, germ, and the endosperm. Each of these components contains various benefits, but many people only consume one of these components of the grain rather than all three.

The bran is an incredibly beneficial aspect of the grain. This portion of the grain contains a large amount of fiber, which aids in regulating digestion, stabilizing blood sugar to prevent spikes or lows, increasing nutrient absorption, reduces the formation of deadly blood clots, increasing satiety, and removing cholesterol from the blood. This component of the grain also contains a large number of other nutrients such as magnesium, iron, zinc, copper, B vitamins, antioxidants, and phytonutrients.

Similarly, the germ has many health benefits as well. This portion of the grain contains important vitamin E and B vitamins as well as antioxidants, phytonutrients, and healthy polyunsaturated fats. The number of antioxidants, phytonutrients, and vitamins within this portion of the grain help fight against disease and aging.

Lastly, the innermost layer of the grain is the endosperm. This portion of the grain holds most of the carbohydrates, protein, and a few other nutrients. The nutrients within the endosperm include B vitamins, magnesium, copper, selenium, and phytonutrients. While this is beneficial, it does not compare to the number of nutrients found within the bran and the germ of the plants.

Sadly, ever since the nineteenth-century grains have become highly processed so that the most nutritious aspects are removed and only the endosperm remains. Due to the most fiber-rich portions of the grain being removed, it causes a spike in blood sugar and loses the many benefits fiber provides. The grains also lose out on most of the vitamins, minerals, antioxidants, and phytonutrients when the brain and germ are removed, leaving you with a product virtually lacking in nutrition.

When shopping for grains keep an eye on our which ones are truly whole grains, as studies have revealed that food labeling can be inconsistent leaving foods labeled as "whole grain" often times unhealthy. Don't simply buy a pre-made item because it says "whole-grain" as this could mean it contains some whole grains but others which are not. The products are still likely to contain sugar and other unhealthy ingredients not recommended on the Mediterranean diet, as well.

Try to stick with whole-grain products that only contain Mediterranean-approved ingredients, contain few added ingredients, and ideally have grains within their full form. While milled whole grains certainly have their benefits, it is ideal for your blood sugar to consume grains in their full form without being milled. This allows your body to absorb the sugars from within the grain more slowly without a spike or crash in blood sugar. For instance, you can simply cook whole corn, brown rice, millet, barley, or oats without having them milled first.

Vegetables and Fruits

Fruits, and especially vegetables, are a phenomenally important aspect of the Mediterranean lifestyle. People throughout the Mediterranean eat these with every meal, centering their protein and grain intake on the vegetables they consume. These vegetables are especially helpful on the Mediterranean diet because unlike in Western countries they don't fry them. Instead, these vegetables are most often served steamed, roasted, or served raw. However, this doesn't mean they are lacking in flavor. After being drizzled in olive oil, topped with nuts, seeds, or citrus, spices, and sometimes even accented with cooked whole grains, these vegetables become a treat that you won't be able to get enough of. Vegetables don't have to be boring, they can be bursting with flavor and texture.

There are many options of vegetables you can choose on the Mediterranean diet, in fact, your options are practically limitless. Although, some of the more popular choices include eggplant, artichokes, broccoli, mushrooms, beets, kale, fennel, onions, peppers, zucchini, sweet potatoes, spinach, radishes, shallots, mustard greens, celery, pumpkin, potatoes, carrots, and cucumbers.

Fresh fruits are a wonderful choice when served without added sugars. These fruits should be eaten whole, as fruit drinks and juices contain a large amount of sugar without fiber to balance it out. It's important to also eat fruit in moderation, as the calories and natural sugars within the fruit can quickly add up. However, you can certainly enjoy these fruits fully whether you're accenting your main meal with them, eating them as a snack, or enjoying them for dessert.

Some of the more popular choices of fruit on the Mediterranean diet includes cherries, dates, grapes, apples, figs, peaches, oranges, pears, pomegranates, melons, nectarines, tangerines, strawberries, lemons, tomatoes, olives, and avocados. Yes, olives and avocados are fruits, not vegetables! These two fruits contain a large number of monounsaturated fats that are essential to the Mediterranean diet. You can enjoy them liberally without worrying about natural sugars. However, you want to watch how many calories you are eating of these fruits, as with their high fat content, the number of calories can add up quickly.

When choosing the vegetables and fruits you are eating on a weekly basis try to vary their colors. For instance, you don't want to eat all green or red vegetables. This is because the nutrition that vegetables contain largely varies upon their color due to the phytonutrients within the ingredients. Try to plan a selection for red, orange, yellow, green white, purple, and even black vegetables within your diet on a weekly basis. By eating a variety of ingredients you can better consume all of the nutrients your body requires and attain optimal nutrition.

Green vegetables such as kale, asparagus, cabbage, broccoli, artichokes, spinach, and green peppers are an important part of a healthy diet. Whether a person is on the Mediterranean diet or not they require a large number of these vegetables. These ingredients are linked to improved prevention of certain cancers and heart disease, as well as strong teeth and bones, and healthy red blood cells.

Within certain green vegetables, specifically cruciferous vegetables such as broccoli and Brussels sprouts, you will taste a strong sulfur compound. Some people enjoy this flavor whereas to others it tastes overwhelmingly strong. However, if you can eat these vegetables, they have some great benefits, such as the ability to strengthen the immune system while lowering blood cholesterol levels.

Some green vegetables, such as cruciferous ones, okra, avocados, spinach, and asparagus, contain glutathione. This is one of the strongest antioxidants, which naturally strengthens the immune system, prevents oxidative stress, improves the insulin response, treats respiratory diseases, and more.

Dark leafy greens contain a large amount of folic acid. This particular nutrient can help prevent heart disease by detoxifying the amino acid homocysteine when it becomes overly populated within the bloodstream. If the homocysteine is allowed to be at a high level within the blood, like cholesterol, it can increase the risk of heart disease, stroke, colon cancer, and Alzheimer's disease. Thankfully, folic acid can reduce the levels of this nutrient to their optimal number so that it does not become toxic. Folic acid is also incredibly important for people who are pregnant. In fact, it is recommended that people consume high levels of folic acid months prior to becoming pregnant to help prevent birth defects.

Red vegetables and fruits, such as red pepper and tomatoes, are a staple in the Mediterranean cuisine. These ingredients can protect heart health, reduce the risk of certain cancers, improve urinary tract health, strengthen memory, and more. Red vegetables often contain the antioxidant beta-carotene and vitamin C, which can increase eye health and prevent cellular damage. These ingredients get their red hue from lycopene, which is an antioxidant which protects against breast and prostate cancers, promotes heart health, reduces oxidative stress, protects against sun exposure and sunburn, increases eye health, protects against neurological disorders, and strengthens bones.

You can find a wide selection of red vegetables, such as certain peppers, cabbage, onions, beets, red potatoes, and kidney beans.

Orange and yellow vegetables contain carotenoids, which are the pigments from which they get their beautiful color. These carotenoids are antioxidants which are well-known to promote eye and skin health. However, they can also lower blood cholesterol levels, reduce the risk of stroke, lower the risk of lung cancer, decrease inflammation, and promote heart health. The lutein and zeaxanthin antioxidants within these vegetables compound upon these benefits, especially by promoting increased eye health.

You can enjoy a wide range of orange and yellow vegetables, such as sweet potatoes, butternut squash, carrots, peppers, oranges, yellow summer squash, and more.

Black, blue, and purple vegetables are highly pigmented, which also means that they are full of antioxidants which prevent cancer, fight heart disease, and promotes healthy aging. One of the antioxidants found within these foods is anthocyanin, which is known as a flavonoid. This antioxidant specifically reduces fatigue, increases healing after exercise, boosts the immune system, protects against neurological disorders, increases cognitive function, improves memory, and much more.

You can find many black, blue, and purple fruits and vegetables. Some options are purple cabbage, eggplant, purple or blue potatoes, purple asparagus, black plums, blood oranges, blue corn, purple endive, black and purple carrots, purple sweet potatoes, blood oranges, berries, and purple grapes.

White, brown, and tan vegetables may be lacking in color, but they are not without their own set of benefits. There are many ingredients within this category that boost overall health with fiber, vitamin C, potassium, selenium, folic acid, and phytonutrients.

Some of the most powerful ingredients in this category are garlic and onion. These two ingredients contain allicin, which has been used for hundreds of years to fight cancer in Chinese medicine. This antioxidant can also lower inflammation, decrease muscle pains, decrease cholesterol, and lower high blood pressure. For this reason, it's recommended to consume a large amount of both garlic and onion.

Some other foods in this color category include leeks, mushrooms, potatoes, turnips, cauliflower, white corn, bananas, parsnips, dates, white peaches, and jicama.

Beans and Legumes

You hear about legumes, but what exactly are they? They are the seeds or fruit of plants from a bean, pea, or other plants in the fabaceae plant family. However, there are many plants that fit under this category. In fact, there are over nineteen thousand and five hundred varieties!

These plants are full of soluble fiber, which lowers cholesterol and keeps your digestion regulated. They are a wonderful source of plant-based protein, making them ideal for people looking to cut back on meat and fish. However, legumes and beans are also extremely affordable, making them accessible for people on a budget. Like whole grains, legumes are a source of carbohydrates. However, due to their high fiber content, they have a low glycemic index and won't spike blood sugar or cause it to crash. This will enable you to also manage or prevent diabetes and feel full for a longer period of time.

Legumes are incredibly dense in nutrients. This enables you to get quite a few vitamins, minerals, antioxidants, fiber, and phytonutrients in a relatively small serving. This can be especially helpful if you are watching your calories and attempting to lose weight. Not only that, but people who are hoping to lose weight on the Mediterranean diet will be especially happy to know that legumes can aid in weight loss. A large study by the Journal of the American College of Nutrition analyzed nearly one-thousand and five hundred people over a period of eight years. This study discovered that people who regularly consume legumes had lower body weight, had a smaller waist, and were twenty-two percent less likely to become obese.

Beans can also improve your heart health and decrease your risk of heart-related illness or death. This is especially true when you pair legumes and beans with an already healthy diet and lifestyle, such as the Mediterranean diet. Legumes have been found to lower dangerous LDL cholesterol, blood triglycerides, high blood pressure, and chronic inflammation.

If you are deficient in any vitamins, then legumes may be the answer. Due to their high nutrition content, you can get a large serving of many of your needed nutrients in a single one cup serving. For instance, a cup of lentils contains ninety percent of your needed folate, forty-nine percent of your manganese, eighteen percent of B6, eighteen percent magnesium, thirty-seven percent iron, seventeen percent zinc, and more. This shows that legumes can greatly help in rounding out nutrition you may be missing out on.

However, beans do have antinutrients, which are compounds which block the absorption of some nutrients and can cause stomach upset. You might feel this if beans make you gassy. However, this isn't a reason to avoid beans. Overall, this plant has many benefits for the human body, and should not be neglected. Instead, you can learn some ways of cooking beans which will reduce the number of antinutrients they contain. Of course, you can always eat plain cooked or canned beans, but you can also choose to prepare them further if you wish.

To take full advantage of the nutrients beans have to offer why not try sprouting or fermenting them? It takes a bit of time, but most of the process isn't hands-on and you can go about your day as usual while the beans do their thing.

Sprouting is the more popular method. Typically to sprout legumes you allow them to soak for twenty-four hours before allowing them to sit out in the open air for twelve to twenty-four hours. With this process, you want to rinse them with clean water every four to six hours to ensure they don't go bad, but the process is quite simple. By sprouting your beans, you will find that it will greatly decrease the number of antinutrients while boosting the number of nutrients within them. This will make the beans easier to digest, trigger less of a gas reaction, and will increase your nutrient intake.

Some great examples of legumes include kidney beans, chickpeas, soybeans, lupin beans, lentils, split peas, black beans, and more. It's also worth noting that peanuts are technically a legume, not a nut, as they grow underground and are part of the fabaceae plant family.

Nuts and Seeds

There are many benefits to nuts and seeds, which all of which can be enjoyed on a Mediterranean diet. These ingredients are full of not only vitamins, minerals, and antioxidants, but also flavor and texture. You will find that while these ingredients are certainly well and good on their own as a mid-afternoon snack, they are especially wonderful when added to a selection of vegetable, grain, or fish dishes. However, you should keep in mind that the calories and fat in nuts and seeds can add up much more quickly than you realize. Therefore, if you find your weight stalling then you might want to measure how many you eat to prevent over-consumption.

There are many nutrient-dense nut and seed options. One of the best of these options, which has been greatly researched, is almonds. Why are these so great? They are full of monounsaturated fats, which is the same type of fat found in olive oil and avocados. Almonds also contain a fair amount of polyunsaturated fat, another healthy fat that we mentioned earlier. Because of these heart-healthy fats almonds have been shown to lower bad cholesterol, reduce the risk of heart disease, and increase weight loss. These nuts are also high in fiber, vitamin E, calcium, potassium, magnesium, and phosphorous.

Almonds have become so well-known for its many health benefits to the point that California has now become the number one producer of this nut in the world. This makes almonds easy to purchase, often at a much better price point than other nuts. You can find delicious recipes for these nuts from many cultures, including those within the Mediterranean and throughout Asia. They are extremely versatile and tasty, making them easy to add to any diet.

Hazelnuts, or filberts, may be more expensive than almonds, but they have many benefits of their own which you don't want to miss out on. This nut is full of fiber, folate, vitamin E, manganese, copper, magnesium, thiamine, vitamin B6, iron, and vitamin K. Like almonds, hazelnuts are also made up largely of monounsaturated fats and polyunsaturated fats.

Along with almonds and walnuts, hazelnuts are incredibly popular on the Mediterranean diet. In fact, researchers used these nuts to conduct a study on heart health on the Mediterranean diet with the addition of mixed nuts. This helped the researchers prove that these nuts, when paired with a Mediterranean diet, can greatly reduce the risk of heart disease.

The pine nut comes specifically from the Mediterranean and is often used in the process of making pesto. This is a wonderful way in which to use this ingredient, as the combination of pine nuts, olive oil, and basil makes powerful food rich with nutrients and flavor. Simply pulse these ingredients together and you have the perfect topping for pizza, pasta, cooked grains, or fish.

The pine nut is high in the fat pinoleic acid, which has been shown in studies to release two hormones which reduce appetite and increases weight loss. This nut is also high in fiber, antioxidants, vitamin K, vitamin E, magnesium, phosphorous, zinc, and iron. While hazelnuts and almonds are mostly made up of monounsaturated fats, pine nuts, on the other hand, have nearly twice the amount of polyunsaturated fats than monounsaturated fats.

Pistachios are wonderful for a nutty snack or when you want to add a distinct punch of flavor to a dish you are making. This nut pairs perfectly with a number of Mediterranean dishes, making it quite easy to add into your diet. While nuts are easy to overeat, people are much less likely to overeat pistachios as they take longer to peel and eat, therefore increasing your satiety. Anyone hoping to lose weight can greatly benefit from this. This little green nut is full of vitamin A, vitamin B6, iron, magnesium, vitamin E, fiber, and monounsaturated fats. By enjoying this nut from time to time you can benefit from its ability to lower cholesterol, increase weight loss, improve gut health, and more.

Walnuts are the most powerful nut when it comes to antioxidants, which therefore means that they have an even stronger ability to fight diseases and aging. Researchers have found that this is due to walnuts containing nearly double the number of antioxidants than any other nut, including the well-renowned almonds and hazelnuts. Another reason to add walnuts to your diet is that they contain a large number of polyunsaturated omega-3 oils, unlike most nuts which are mainly comprised of monounsaturated fats. This enables walnuts to balance your omega-3 to omega-6 ratio, in the process lowering inflammation, preventing cancer, and reducing the risk of heart disease. Most people on a Western diet don't consume enough omega-3 fats, making this incredibly beneficial.

There are many nuts you can consume on the Mediterranean diet, but one of the best options is the sesame seed. This is often eaten in the form of tahini, a ground sesame seed paste, which is then added to hummus, eggplant dip, and even Mediterranean sweets! You can easily add these seeds or the paste produced from them to most dishes, sweet or savory.

This tiny little seed is packed full of antioxidants, fiber, calcium, iron, potassium, and magnesium. They also contain other nutrients in a smaller number, such as vitamin E and vitamin B6. This seed is made up largely of both polyunsaturated fats and monounsaturated fats.

I highly recommend adding tahini paste to your diet, it will not only improve the flavor of your dishes but also your health. You can see the evidence of this in studies that have found sesame seeds to manage diabetes, reduce the risk of heart disease, strengthen bone health, boost cellular functioning, lower inflammation, protect against radiation, improve skin and hair health, and the list goes on.

Olive Oil

One of the vital staples of the Mediterranean diet is extra virgin olive oil. Studies have found that this is an incredibly powerful aspect of the Mediterranean diet, as it contributes to a large portion of the weight loss, increased energy, lowered cholesterol, and other health benefits. A study from Spain found that when vegetables are sautéed or roasted in olive oil they contain many more antioxidants and other nutrient compounds known as phenols than vegetables cooked with other methods. It's also important to note that there are many vitamins, such as vitamin A, which are fat soluble and unable to be absorbed without being combined with fat. This means that if you eat a salad or other vegetables with a fat-free dressing you are likely missing out on certain vitamins. By simply drizzling some olive oil over your meal you can ensure you absorb all of the nutrients your body requires.

However, you can enjoy extra virgin olive oil in more ways than on just vegetables. This staple is used for nearly everything throughout the Mediterranean. Citrus salad, sauces, soups, means, seafood, fish, pasta, even desserts are made with olive oil! This oil is wonderful for you, tastes great, and goes with just about anything.

While you want to use olive oil frequently, you need to be careful to buy the correct variety. Not all olive oil is created equally. The first thing you want to check for is that it's extra virgin olive oil. This type of olive oil is created when the fruit of the olive is fully crushed, separated to remove the solids, and then once again separated so that the water is removed from the oil. Non-extra virgin olive oils use heat and chemicals to separate the oil from the fruit, which results in it killing off the powerful nutrients. This oil then goes through a rigorous testing process with global standards that are set by the International Olive Council. The testing process includes official lab testing which tests acidity levels, along with other measurements, as well as a sensory test. The sensory test is completed by a professionally trained olive oil taster to ensure it meets a high-quality standard.

When olive oil doesn't pass this test or has been purified with heat or chemicals then it won't have a seal certifying it as being extra virgin olive oil. This won't have the same health benefits and is sold either as plain olive oil or is labeled as plain, classic, light, or extra light. While these versions of olive oil are less expensive, you won't be able to acquire all of the benefits from the Mediterranean diet with them. Instead, stick with truly extra virgin olive oil.

Although, just because olive oil passed this test doesn't mean it's high quality. There are a few other things you should check for. Olive oil isn't non-perishable, and because of this it can degrade overtime if exposed to light, hear, or air. To prevent from buying low-quality extra virgin olive oil look for a bottle that's sold in a dark bottle or tin to limit the amount of light exposure. After purchase store it in a cabinet that's dark and away from the oven so that the heat or light doesn't damage it.

You will want to check the best by date on the bottle of the oil. You want it to have a date that is at least a year away, which should ensure that it's been bottled within the previous year since they are usually sold for up to two years after bottling. Some brands might even have a harvest date for the olives, which will further ensure you get the best product. Lastly, never buy more than you can use within two months.

Spices

There are many reasons to add spices to your food. While most people only think of these as a way to add flavors and aroma, there is much more reason to add these ingredients. Firstly, by adding spices you can cut down on your sodium intake, which is especially helpful for those with a heart condition or diabetes. However, what most people don't realize is that these spices have many beneficial phytonutrients and effects. After all, these same spices and herbs have been used for centuries to treat disease.

Parsley is bright and fresh, with the ability to be added to practically anything. Do you have soup? Top it with parsley. Want to brighten a salad? Add parsley. Want a refreshing sauce from some fish? Make a chimichurri sauce. There are endless options when it comes to parsley. This herb also contains many vitamins, anti-inflammatory properties, promotes better digestion, strengthens bones, treats bladder infections, freshens breath, protects eye health, and more.

Thyme is another popular herb with many uses. This herb is especially helpful when used to brighten bean, vegetable, fish, or poultry dishes. This herb is microbial, boosts the immune system, lessens sore throats, lowers high blood pressure and cholesterol, boosts mood, fights cancer, treats coughs, and helps to prevent contamination from food poisoning.

You can use basil, dry or fresh, in a variety of dishes. Try to always keep some dried leaves in your pantry, but it is even better if you grow some in a pot to always have fresh on hand. This will ensure you can always use the fresh herb to accent a dish without paying an arm and a leg. If you are someone who especially loves basil, then you might want to grow several pots of the plant so that you have enough to make pesto and Caprese salad. Some of the benefits of basil include blood cell protection, boosting the immune system, reducing inflammation, relieving stress, reducing fevers, protecting the liver, and it can even relieve pain!

Rosemary has a pleasant pine and floral flavor that can highlight poultry, soups and stews, and root vegetables deliciously. Although, it can accent many other dishes, as well. This herb is tenacious and hardy, easy to grow in a pot or in the ground. Along with all the good flavor accompanying this spice, you will also gain improved brain health, pain relief, less stress, increased circulation, reduced inflammation, and more.

Cilantro is fresh and bright, absolutely vital for most Mexican and Indian dishes. Although for some people this refreshing herb tastes like soap, so they might want to replace it with parsley. It won't have the same taste, but it is usually the best alternative. Along with its powerful flavor, cilantro has a powerful ability to detoxify the body from heavy metals, improve sleep, reduce anxiety, fights against oxidative stress, lowers high blood sugar, protects against cardiovascular disease, treats urinary tract infections, prevents inflammation in the brain, increases skin health, and more.

Saffron is expensive, one of the most expensive spices, but you don't require much of it to kick up a dish to the next level. Best yet, this spice is used traditionally in Mediterranean cooking and will greatly expand the number of dishes you can try out in the kitchen. This spice, which is a flower, is an antioxidant, lifts the mood, lowers appetite, increases weight loss, fights cancer, reduces the risk of heart disease, and may lessen the symptoms of Alzheimer's disease with its antioxidant effects.

Lastly, you might look for za'atar spice blend. The exact benefits of this blend depend upon the recipe or brand, as it will change depending upon the ingredients. However, it contains many herbs and spices that have beneficial effects. In this blend, you can often find oregano, thyme, and marjoram. Sometimes, salt, dried sumac, or sesame seeds may even be added.

There are many other foods you can enjoy within the Mediterranean food pyramid. However, if you focus on the ingredients mentioned here, then you can add in the other ingredients such as seafood, poultry, and dairy—and you'll be okay. Remember, there are multiple tiers of the Mediterranean food pyramid, but you want to keep the second tier, the first of the food tiers after staying athletic, as your main focus.

Chapter 6: How to Easily Transform Your Lifestyle for Better Health

The Mediterranean diet is not only a diet but an entire lifestyle. However, changing your life and adopting a new lifestyle can be daunting. Sure, all the knowledge you have been provided within this book hands you the knowledge and tools you require, but you still have to make the change.

Don't fear. Within this chapter, you will be provided with tips, tricks, and plans to help you more easily adopt the Mediterranean lifestyle and better health. If you are someone who is always motivated to make lifestyle changes and never hesitates, you might decide to jump right in—and that's perfectly fine! On the other hand, if you are someone who prefers to dip your toes into the pool before diving in, then you will find this chapter incredibly helpful and beneficial. There's no reason to let a better life, better health, and good food scare you into hesitation. I will walk through the process with you—making the Mediterranean lifestyle simple and natural.

Switch Fats

One of the simplest changes you can make when beginning the Mediterranean diet is switching the sources of fat you use. You likely already buy and cook with fat, whether it's butter, vegetable oil, canola oil, lard, or a number of other fats. Instead of choosing these fats with few health benefits and unhealthy fatty acids, such as saturated fatty acids, you can replace them with something better. When choosing fat, you always want to use extra virgin olive oil—not classic or light-tasting olive oil but extra virgin. As we mentioned earlier, other versions of olive oil do not contain all of the same vital nutrients, which is what makes this type of fat so powerful.

Whether you are cooking vegetables, toasting bread, or cooking an entire meal, you can use extra virgin olive oil in place of other fats. This is an easy and inexpensive way to make a lifestyle change, as you will simply replace the other sources of fat you had been buying with a new source of fat.

Make a Dairy Change

Dairy, like most animal-based products, ids high in saturated fats. These are fats that can increase inflammation and decrease your overall health. While you don't have to refrain from animal-based products completely, you do want to make better choices. One way in which you can easily make better dairy choices is by switching to a low-fat version of dairy, as this will greatly decrease the number of saturated fats you are consuming.

For instance, one cup of whole milk contains four and a half grams of saturated fats, while one percent of milk only contains one and a half grams. One cup of whole-fat mozzarella cheese contains fifteen grams of saturated fat, yet the low-fat version contains a much lower number of three grams.

The same applies to yogurt. While you can certainly enjoy yogurt, especially Greek yogurt, on the Mediterranean diet, stick to low-fat or fat-free versions. Many brands sell fat-free versions of Greek yogurt, which obviously contain no saturated fats. However, other brands sell five-percent-fat versions of Greek yogurt, which contain an entire eight grams for one single cup of yogurt. This is almost twice the amount of saturated fat found in an equal amount of whole milk! By simply changing the type of dairy you choose you can greatly benefit your health and make a steady change toward a complete Mediterranean lifestyle.

However, remember that dairy is still a limited ingredient on the Mediterranean food pyramid. You can certainly enjoy these ingredients multiple times a week, but try to limit it to no more than once a day.

Replace Red Meat with Fish

You don't have to completely replace meat or red meat with fish. Although, try to lower the amount of red meat you are consuming while replacing at least two of your meat dishes with fish a week. Ideally, you want this fish to be a fatty fish such as salmon or sardines so that you can consume all of the important omega-3 fatty acids your body requires. Not will this change just increase the amount of omega-3 you are eating, it will also further limit the number of saturated fats you are consuming. This is a win-win, allowing you to improve your health on multiple fronts by making a single change. While you don't have to completely cut out red meat, you want to highly limit it. When you do treat yourself and allow yourself to have some, try to stick with lower-fat cuts to reduce the number of saturated fats you are eating.

If you feel like eating meat one night but aren't in the mood to eat fish, you can always eat poultry. Whether chicken, duck, or another source of poultry, there are many ways in which you can cook and flavor these ingredients. However, you will still want to choose lower-fat options of poultry when possible, as this still contains saturated fats. Poultry does contain less saturated fat than red meat, but it's still there and you need to be careful of the amount you are consuming. While one cup of chicken breast contains only one and a half grams of saturated fat, the same amount of chicken thighs contains over twice that.

Increase Your Fruit and Vegetable Intake

Fruits and vegetables are one of the most important components of the Mediterranean diet, along with other plant-based foods. However, most Americans and others on the Western diet don't consume the minimum recommendation of these vital foods. This has been shown to lead to an increase in not only weight but disease and mortality risk. Simply by increasing the number of plant-based foods within your diet, you can greatly increase your health, weight loss, and adherence to the Mediterranean lifestyle. However, this is easier said than done for many people. Most people on the Western diet live off of the occasional vegetable that might show up on their pizza or next to their steak. However, don't worry, there are a few ways you can easily increase your vegetable and fruit intake.

One of the ways in which you can increase your vegetable and fruit intake is simply by replacing some of the junk food you buy with plant-based ingredients. This may sound obvious, but if you stock your pantry with ice cream and cookies and only a couple vegetables or fruits, which are you more likely to reach for? Therefore, when shopping, don't reach for the unneeded junk food snacks and instead pick out vegetables and fruits that are easy to eat quickly for snacks. This way, if you find yourself craving something sweet at night you are more likely to reach for some fruit than a cookie.

You might even begin to make a game of how many fruits and vegetables you can eat. Eating breakfast? Consider what vegetables might taste good in an omelet or which fruits on yogurt. If you are making dinner, consider all the vegetable options and try to find one you can include. Maybe you decide to make baked sweet potato fries or sautéed asparagus with garlic. Once you get in the habit of challenging yourself to include fruits and vegetables in every meal you will find it becomes second nature.

Make cooking with fruits and vegetables as easy as possible. I don't know about you, but when I've had a long day I don't want to spend a long time in the kitchen. However, if immediately after grocery shopping you wash, chop, and store your produce you can easily grab it with little effort. If you already have chopped asparagus, cherry tomatoes, and minced garlic in the fridge then you can easily toss them in the oven with some olive oil. Once they are done cooking you can place them on salad, with wild or brown rice, toss them in pasta, really the choices are endless. This will enable you to greatly increase the number of fruits and vegetables you eat with minimal effort.

Lastly, if you already have fruits and vegetables prepared in the fridge and freezer you can prepare a quick breakfast or snack on-the-go by making a smoothie. Your smoothie doesn't only have to include fruits, even! You can toss in spinach, kale, celery, avocado, and many other vegetables for a boost in nutrition. Try adding in plant-based protein or egg white protein powders, chia seeds, ground flax seeds, tahini paste, matcha powder, olive oil, and other healthy-boosting ingredients for an even better meal.

Boost Your Whole-Grain Intake

Whole grains are infinitely healthier, more filling, and more nutritious than their highly-processed brethren. Try to slowly boost your whole-grain intake while you are diminishing your processed grain intake. By doing this you will increase the nutrients you are consuming, improve your health, stay fuller and satisfied for longer periods of time, and more. However, many people are unsure how to increase their whole-grain

86

intake in more ways than simply switching to whole-grain bread. Let me tell you, switching to whole-grain bread is a great start, but there are other easy tips you can use as well.

Firstly, you can begin by switching to the whole-grain version of foods you already eat. This doesn't just include bread, but also pasta, rice, flour, and more. When going shopping see if any of the grain products you regularly consume come in whole-grain varieties. However, don't be fooled into clever marketing that is meant to trick the consumer. Legally, within America any product labeled as "whole grain" must consume at least eight grams of whole grains and all of the grains within it must be whole and minimally processed. However, some companies label their products as "multigrain" or "natural" in order to get more sales from health-conscious people. The problem is that multigrain doesn't mean that the product has any added nutrition, only that it contains more than one type of grain, even if it is highly processed. "Natural" is an even more dubious claim, as this label contains no meaning. The FDA allows anyone to label their products as "natural," as it is not an official label. Therefore, make sure that the product specifically says "whole grain" and contains the grains within the first three ingredients on the label.

If you are used to snacking on potato chips and pretzels as snacks you might not know what to do to get your savory fix. While you could always make homemade baked fries, sometimes you want something with grains and that is more portable. The good news is that popcorn is a whole grain and can be cooked well in advance! If you are having a movie night or hope to take a snack to work simply pop some corn and then toss it in some olive oil and your favorite seasonings. You will find that this is much tastier than microwave varieties and still quite simple!

Lastly, don't be afraid to try new things. Quinoa has become popular in recent years, but there are many other grains to choose from as well. Why not try wild rice, millet, farro, bulgur, sorghum, spelt, kamut, and teff? These grains, like rice, are simple to cook. However, they all offer a variety of nutrition and flavor.

Don't Miss Out on Breakfast

Studies have shown that people who skip breakfast are more likely to overeat later. This is because the body knows it needs to eat, therefore even if they didn't feel hungry in the morning, by evening they will feel the intense urge to eat. This causes many people to not only eat too much food but often eating the wrong types of food. Often times in this situation a person will grab whatever food is easy and that they are craving, whether its doughnuts, pizza, French fries, or Chinese takeout. Even if you skip breakfast hoping to reduce your calorie intake and shed some pounds, it is often better for your weight loss and calorie count to instead eat a small healthy breakfast.

By eating nutrient-dense foods such as whole grains, yogurt, eggs, fruits, and vegetables you can stay full for longer and reduce junk food cravings exponentially.

Practice Cooking Vegetarian

While the Mediterranean diet isn't a vegetarian or vegan diet, it does prioritize plant-based ingredients. The main tier of the Mediterranean pyramid consists of grains, vegetables, fruits, legumes, beans, nuts, seeds, spices, and olive oil. Therefore, try to have meatless meals that are made up of these ingredients. This will help you to learn to better use plant-based proteins and ingredients, making your life easier in the future. You will also find having a vegetarian meal or day, such as Meatless Monday, will boost your nutrition and overall health. Before long you will find that cooking vegetarian meals is quite simple on the Mediterranean diet, as there is an enormous amount of ingredients you can choose to cook with. For instance, why not make a pasta or farro dish with some beans, nuts, vegetables, and of course some olive oil and your favorite seasonings? By doing this you can have an endless variety of flavor options, yet always know of an easy and simple meatless dish to cook.

Choose Fish Wisely

There are many reasons to include fish in your diet, especially fatty fish which are rich in omega-3 fatty acids. However, it's important to know that almost all fish and seafood contain traces of the toxic element mercury. If you eat too much fish that is high in this substance it can greatly damage your health. Therefore, it's important to know which fish are more likely to contain higher amounts of mercury and what your best options include.

One of the best tricks to limiting the amount of mercury you eat is by consuming smaller fish. Larger fish naturally eat smaller fish in nature, which results in the larger fish not only containing its own mercury but absorbing the mercury that was in the smaller fish it ate. This adds up over time as big fish continue to eat small fish. However, small fish usually don't eat other fish, resulting in a much lower mercury level. Try to limit fish such as tuna, swordfish, shark, and king mackerel.

The National Defense Research Council recommends eating halibut, sea bass, albacore and yellowfin tuna, white pacific croaker, ocean perch, sablefish, and gulf or Spanish mackerel no more than three times every month.

Shark, swordfish, bluefish, king mackerel, bigeye and ahi tuna, marlin, grouper, and orange roughly are completely recommended against by the National Defense Research Council or NDRC.

The NDRC recommends eating bass, crab, tuna (Canned chunk light, Skipjack), snapper, Atlantic tilefish, freshwater perch, mahi-mahi, monkfish, buffalo fish, carp, sheepshead, and Alaskan cod no more than six times each month.

There are many kinds of fish on the frequently enjoyed list by the NDRC, but some of the most common include salmon, tilapia, anchovies, catfish, herring, oysters, freshwater trout, sardines, shrimp, crawfish, sole, calamari, flounder, and scallops.

You might also want to keep an eye out on fish advisories online so that you can be aware of any contamination or concerns that are important to know of. This can be important, as sometimes fish, such as tilapia, are farmed in poor condition which leads to health concerns. For this reason, it's also often best to choose wild-caught fish varieties rather than farm-raised. You will be charged a little more, but wild-caught fish have many more nutrients and much more flavor.

Children who are younger than twelve and people who are either pregnant or nursing should only eat fish from the low-mercury list. While the moderate mercury list which contains fish such as mahi-mahi and crab can be enjoyed from time to time by other people, it could interfere with the development and growth of children. This is why it shouldn't only be avoided by children themselves, but also those who are pregnant or nursing.

Keep an Eye on the Food Pyramid

It helps to print out a copy of the Mediterranean food pyramid and keep it in your kitchen so you can view it with a glance whenever you are cooking or planning your menu. The food pyramid by Old Ways is the most commonly used Mediterranean food pyramid and easily found online.

By having the pyramid in plain view you will be easily able to get food and meal ideas, but more importantly, you can ensure you eat correctly. Most Americans are used to the USDA's food pyramid, which is quite different from the Mediterranean version. For instance, the

The Mediterranean food pyramid, unlike the USDA's version, emphasizes the importance of healthy fats, limited red meat, and sweets (including sugar-heavy fruits), and dairy is not as heavily recommended.

Eat and Cook with Family or Friends

The bottom and first tier of the Mediterranean food pyramid emphasizes the importance of an active life and enjoying meals with loved ones. While we may not be able to eat every meal with someone we care about, and this is much more limited for those who live alone, try to eat with others when you get the chance. It could be a family member, friend, a date, or even a coworker.

Why worry about this? It has been shown that by eating with others we are much less likely to overeat as we eat slowly while talking. In turn, this will increase weight loss and reduce the number of excess calories you may be eating. By eating slowly, you can also improve your digestion of the meal.

You will find that instead of eating in front of the TV, computer, or with a smartphone in hand, your mental health will get a boost by eating with another person. Stress will be released, making following the Mediterranean diet over the following days easier to manage.

It is common in many cultures throughout the world for people to get together to share food and drinks. The experience of sharing a meal together both strengthens the enjoyment of the food and adds spice to the company. However, it has become increasingly common in our modern Western society for people to skip out on eating meals together when busy. Even more frequently families aren't sharing a meal together, and when they do it is in front of the TV or with cell phones in hand.

Try to challenge yourself to eat more with others. If you have a family try setting aside at least one night a week where you all share a meal, without electronics. If you are someone unable to eat with their family, then try to find friends or coworkers who you can begin inviting over for meals or going out to eat with. However, if you choose to go out to eat ensure that the food you eat is still healthy and fits within the Mediterranean diet pyramid.

Get a Sweat Worked Up

Yes, it's hard to make time to work out when you lead a busy life. For this reason, gyms are able to make quite a bit of money off of people who sign up for a membership at the beginning of the year, yet never actually go. However, whether you choose to purchase a gym membership or not it's vital for your health to exercise frequently and work up a sweat. No matter your gender, age, or physical ability, exercise is necessary for health.

One of the most important aspects of exercise is that it prevents disease and slows down aging. Many of the most common killers in America, such as heart disease, high cholesterol, high blood pressure, cancer, metabolic syndrome, depression, Alzheimer's disease, and others can be at the very least improved with regular exercise. You may be able to reduce your risk of developing these conditions, help manage and treat them, or even prevent them altogether if you exercise regularly.

If you are hoping that the Mediterranean diet will help you to lose weight that is even more reason to practice exercise. Combined with a healthy diet, specifically this diet, exercise can increase the burning of fat and boost metabolism. You don't have to exercise for long periods, but if you work up a sweat for twenty to thirty minutes a few days a week then you will be well on your way to a healthier weight.

Many people in today's society are short on energy from living always on the go, eating poorly, and sleeping less. However, this can be combated with exercise. While exercise may decrease your energy immediately after the fact in the beginning, you will find that over time it strengthens your endurance, strength, and heart health, giving you more energy for the things you want. This boost in endorphins from exercise can also provide you with a burst of energy and stamina.

Exercise can even improve your mood, which is increasingly important with the number of people with depression, anxiety, and other mental illnesses on the rise. While medication and therapy may help these conditions, they often are not enough alone. By treating your mental health with a full lifestyle approach, including exercise and diet, you will find that you feel more relaxed, less depressed, and less anxious. You may even find that your confidence and self-esteem increase.

If you find yourself frequently tossing and turning at night, unable to fall asleep, unable to stay asleep, or simply sleeping lightly, then excise can help. Exercise has been proven to help people both fall asleep and stay asleep better.

Lastly, many people will be happy to know that by increasing their exercise they can boost their sex life and bring more spice back into the bedroom. This is because as you get into better shape you will not only look better, but with your increased energy, strength, and flexibility you will be able to have more fun.

However, just because you are prioritizing exercise doesn't mean you can't have fun. Take a spin or yoga class, take up dancing, find a local group to play sports with, take up hiking, go biking or skating with your kids, why not try canoeing? Whatever you choose you can have fun. Try to give yourself twenty to thirty minutes to exercise five to six days a week. Although, if you choose to participate in vigorous exercise you can cut it down to only three times a week.

As you can see, there are many small steps you can take in order to adopt the Mediterranean lifestyle. It may seem overwhelming at first, but if you take the process in steps you will find it much more natural and easier. If you desire you can try adopting one of these steps each week until you are completing all of them. Or, you can even choose to take multiple steps written about within this chapter at a time. Whatever you choose, be sure that you take the time you need and adopt the Mediterranean diet at your own speed.

Chapter 7: Frequently Asked Questions and Answers for Success

There are many questions people have about the Mediterranean diet. Some of these questions may have already been answered throughout this book, but this chapter seeks to answer the most asked questions. You can use this chapter as a quick answer guide prior to reading the book to help yourself answer questions from family members—or even after reading the book to brush up on what you have learned. In whatever means that you use this section, there are sure to be some questions you want answers to, and we seek to answer as many as we can here.

Can I Have Carbs on the Mediterranean Diet?

You may be wondering about carbs or carbohydrates. This is especially true after the popularity of the Atkins and now Ketogenic diets, which both extremely limit the intake of carbs. People assume that carbs make you gain weight, simply because carbohydrates lead to a small amount of water weight. The problem is that this water weight doesn't affect your health and is quite small, so it's not something that should be feared. More than that, carbohydrates are important for energy.

Lastly, there is a difference between healthy carbs and unhealthy carbs. Yes, carbs from highly processed white bread, cereals, corn syrup, sugar, and other junk food is incredibly unhealthy and unnecessary. On the other hand, whole grains, vegetables, fruits, legumes, and nuts all contain healthy sources of carbohydrates which are full of nutrients and fiber.

The Mediterranean diet doesn't seek to limit these foods, as countless research has found them to be incredibly beneficial for not only overall health and the prevention of disease but also weight loss for those who are concerned.

There is nothing wrong with eating pasta or bread in moderation. These foods are eaten widely across the Mediterranean without ill effects on health or weight. Why is this? Because in the Mediterranean pasta and bread are eaten in small servings alongside many other ingredients, such as vegetables, legumes, and fish. This is what the Mediterranean diet seeks to emulate.

Can I Have Meat on the Mediterranean Diet?

Yes, you can have meat! Being on the Mediterranean diet doesn't mean you also have to be vegetarian or vegan, although you can choose to be if you desire. However, meat is eaten in much smaller portions on the Mediterranean diet than on the standard Western diet. For instance, you may only eat red meat once a week. Although, you can still have other forms of meat. You might have both fish and poultry throughout your week to complement your meals. These types of meat have many benefits and include much less saturated fats.

When you do buy red meat, while only an occasional treat, try to buy higher quality meat with less fat. If you can afford beef without antibiotics, hormones, and grass-fed it will have many more health benefits than cheaper red meat. By choosing a low-fat cut of red meat you can decrease the number of saturated fats you are eating.

What If I Don't Have Time to Cook?

It's not always easy to fit cooking into our busy lives, especially if we work a job with long hours. However, it's important to prioritize your health and therefore cooking. Thankfully there are many ways in which you can cut down on the time it takes to prepare food.

For instance, you can keep some whole-wheat pasta and bread on hand. With these, you can easily add a number of ingredients for a complete meal. Some options might be frozen fish fillets which only take a few moments to cook, frozen vegetable steam bags, canned beans, store-bought hummus, or pre-chopped fruits and vegetables from the produce department. There are many ways in which you can cut down on time in the kitchen by purchasing pre-made or ingredients which cook quickly with little effort. You may also decrease the time it takes to cook by immediately preparing ingredients when you get home from the grocery store. Cook pasta or rice to store in the fridge, wash and chop your vegetables, roast some chicken, there are endless options to create simple and quick meals on the Mediterranean diet.

What Do I Shop for on the Mediterranean Diet?

Olive Oil: Buy plenty of extra virgin olive oil. You don't want "classic," "pure," "light-tasting," or "extra light" olive oil, as these have been overly processed, sometimes using chemicals and heat, and do not contain the same amount of health benefits. Olive oil will be your main source of fat on the Mediterranean diet.

Whole Grains: You want to buy whole grains and cereals, such as whole-wheat bread and pasta, brown rice wild rice, farro, millet, teff, barley, quinoa, couscous, and others. There are many delicious grains you can try that have a number of nutrients and a large amount of fiber.

Legumes: Buying legumes, specifically beans, and lentils is a great way to get a meatless protein source. Not only that, but legumes have been proven to have many nutritional benefits. You will find that by including more beans and lentils in your diet you can stay full for longer and have more meal options.

Vegetables: Try to buy as many fresh vegetables as you can, and if the selection in the produce department doesn't look too good you can switch to frozen. Some people may also simply prefer frozen vegetables as they don't spoil quickly and are already prepped and ready to use. However, try to stay away from canned vegetables other than beans.

Fish: Buy healthy fish that are low in mercury. Ideally, you want to buy fish that contain a larger amount of fat, such as salmon and sardines, as these contain more of the beneficial omega-3 fatty acids. If you are buying your fish freshly get them from a fishmonger rather than the grocery store. However, these will have to be used immediately so that they don't go bad.

Otherwise, you can find frozen fillets which store for a long period of time in the freezer.

Does the Mediterranean Diet Have Smoothies?

If you like smoothies, then they can be a great way to add more fruits and vegetables to your diet. However, it's important to be careful with smoothies. Yes, they are healthy. However, smoothies pack in a large number of calories and sugars in a single drink. The sugar may originate from fruit, but that doesn't matter, because it is still sugar. Therefore, keep smoothies as an occasional treat and limit the amount of fruit you add.

Can I Have Starbucks Coffee?

The Mediterranean is definitely okay on the Mediterranean diet! In fact, some of the countries that border the Mediterranean are well-known for their coffee. Although, you have to be careful of your coffee order.

The easiest way to get coffee at Starbucks is to order a plain cup of black coffee or espresso. With this order, you can get your caffeine fix without unnecessary ingredients. However, if you are someone who goes to Starbucks specifically for the "unnecessary" ingredients that they add to your coffee, then this may not appeal to you. Don't fear, there are still other options.

You will want to avoid any of the Starbucks flavored drinks, whole milk, and whipped cream. However, you can still enjoy an un-flavored cappuccino, Frappuccino, latte, or flat white. Order these with low-fat, non-fat, or dairy-free kinds of milk.

Along with coffee, you may also order an unflavored matcha latte or tea.

What Is the Mediterranean Diet Based On?

The Mediterranean diet is based on the diet of the Greece island of Crete prior to the addition of junk food within their diet after the 1960s. Studies on this island and other Mediterranean countries have found that there is an incredible benefit to both health and weight when following this diet. The reason for this is multifaceted, but it is largely due to the incorporation of olive oil, a high consumption rate of many antioxidants, low rate of saturated fat consumption, no junk food, and a healthy balance between various food groups.

Is There a Right Way to Follow the Diet?

There are many "right" ways you can follow the Mediterranean diet. Just because two people's journeys on the Mediterranean diet look different doesn't mean that one of them is wrong. For instance, one person may be on a vegan Mediterranean diet while another person is on a more classic Mediterranean diet. One person may stick to strict Mediterranean recipes, while another person follows the Mediterranean pyramid while cooking dishes from various cultures. One person may make all their food from scratch while yet another person takes shortcuts by using frozen vegetables and previously prepared ingredients.

None of these people are wrong in the way they are following the Mediterranean diet. Of course, there are wrong ways you can follow the lifestyle. For instance, if someone drinks sodas it's not a true Mediterranean diet. It may have health benefits for them, but it doesn't fit within the Mediterranean food pyramid.

The Mediterranean Diet Uses Olives, Avocados, and Nuts—What About the Fat Content?

The Western world has had a war on fat for a few decades now. For a long time, "low-fat" was popular and anything that wasn't low in fat was seen as detrimental to overall health, heart health, and weight loss. However, thankfully overtime this misconception has been overturned. Researchers have now proven that it isn't fat itself that is negatively impactful, but the types of fat you eat and how much.

In high concentration, anything will cause you to lose weight. This includes fat, especially because it is high in calories. However, if you watch how much you are eating and aren't needlessly piling on extra fat over your needed caloric intake then you should be fine.

Secondly, the fats used in the Mediterranean diet are some of the healthiest fats known to man. While the Mediterranean diet promotes the use of these powerful fats, it also limits the number of unhealthy fats you eat. For instance, you won't consume much trans-fat on the Mediterranean diet.

Because of this, the Mediterranean diet has been proven to lower blood cholesterol, lower triglycerides, blood sugar, body weight, and the risk of developing or dying from heart disease.

Remember, not all fats are created equal.

Chapter 8: Two-Week Meal Plan to Get You on Your Way

There are many reasons to plan your week ahead when attempting to go on the Mediterranean diet—or any other healthy lifestyle, for that matter—although the three main reasons are time, money, and health. In this chapter, we will go over the importance of planning ahead. You will also get a head start by being provided with a complete and ready-to-go two-week menu plan. With this plan, you can get started on the Mediterranean diet right away with confidence in yourself.

The first of the three reasons to plan ahead, time, is especially important in our modern society. Nearly everyone is always on the go between work, family, social lives, medical care, transportation time, home management, pets, and more. Sometimes, it can be difficult to get a single spare moment. However, if you are trying to eat healthily you are unable to simply go through the drive-through and grab whatever combo of greasy burger and fries is available. Therefore, you must make eating healthy as time efficient as possible so that it can fit within your life in a maintainable manner. This is where meal planning comes in. By planning ahead, you can prepare meals ahead of time for busy days of the week, pack meals to go on the road, or even have meals ready in the freezer for you and your family.

Not only can planning ahead save you time when it comes to eating, but you can also save time in the cooking and shopping process. One great example of this is that you can easily shop only once a week. Think about it, if you don't plan ahead of time you are likely to run out of foods you need throughout the week, leading to multiple spontaneous shopping trips. On the other hand, if you know exactly what you are going to eat you can buy everything you will need and limit your shopping to one day.

If you are unsure what you will eat for the week you are also more likely to aimlessly walk around the grocery store. You look for what you are going to eat, not sure what to buy. At the time this may not seem wasteful, but this can suck up your time more quickly than you notice.

When you are planning ahead you might decide to go ahead and prep some of your meals or ingredients ahead to save time, as well. For instance, if you are chopping onions, garlic, broccoli, or other ingredients and know you will need later on in the week you might as well chop enough for both occasions. You can use what you need at the moment and store the rest in the fridge so you don't have to waste time chopping and cleaning up again. Thinking ahead and little actions such as this can be big time savers.

If you don't mind eating the same dish multiple times a week you can plan to make fewer but larger dishes, so that you can eat leftovers multiple times. This can be extremely helpful, especially if you are a person who frequently feels too worn out to cook. On the way home and too tired to cook while feeling tempted to just grab fast food? No need to feel that temptation, as you will have a delicious meal already fully cooked in the fridge or freezer.

Like many people, you might not be a morning person. If that's the case, then you can especially be helped out by a healthy Mediterranean breakfast ready to go. I don't know about you, but the first thing I want to do every morning is to get coffee, and the last thing I want is to cook. However, with a little forethought, you can have the filling and satisfying nutrition you need without having to think or move much before the caffeine kicks in.

Lastly, if you are someone who's always having to go out to grab something to eat during your lunch break at work, you can gain more time for yourself. Instead of spending your precious break rushing to get food in time to eat it, you can have a healthy meal ready and packed to take to work with you and leisurely enjoy.

Eating out and buying junk food can become incredibly expensive. On the other hand, it has been shown that by cooking your own meals you can save money. Sure, some healthy ingredients may be more expensive. However, by planning ahead you can find healthy ingredients that are approved on the Mediterranean diet at a fair and accessible price.

Food waste is also money waste. Many people will keep their fridges stocked with the food they hope to eat, such as spinach, kale, fish, and yogurt. However, since they never planned how they were going to use these ingredients before they bought them they often go to waste. However, when you plan ahead you only buy what you need, eliminating this waste and saving you money. This is not only better for your wallet but better for the environment, as well.

For people who are especially tight on funds, you can check the sale papers and coupons when planning. This will allow you to find healthy Mediterranean diet friendly ingredients that are at a discount. For instance, you may look to see if any canned, frozen, or fresh produce is on sale. Maybe a store is having a discount on whole rice or dried beans. Various seafood and dairy products frequently go on sale, as well.

Week One

Sunday

Breakfast: Scrambled eggs with olive oil, cherry tomatoes, spinach, basil, and feta cheese.

Lunch: Whole-wheat pita bread filled with chickpea salad made with chickpeas, tahini, Dijon mustard, apple cider vinegar, olive oil, and capers. Can also add tomatoes, olives, and basil to the pita, as well.

Snack: Endive filled with herb goat cheese, dill, and smoked salmon.

Dinner: Penne pasta with shrimp, lemon, olive oil, basil, Parmesan, and sun-dried tomatoes.

Monday

Breakfast: Greek yoghurt with honey, walnuts, and sliced banana.

Lunch: Whole-wheat bun with a turkey burger, lettuce, tomato, and Tzatziki sauce.

Snack: Chickpea salad with fresh tomatoes, olives, cucumber, parsley, basil, feta, lemon juice, and olive oil.

Dinner: Roasted chicken, potatoes, carrots, and beets with olive oil and rosemary.

Tuesday

Breakfast: Whole-grain toast topped with tahini and fruit of choice.

Lunch: Vegetable risotto with garlic, olive oil, bail, red onion, and roasted tomatoes, zucchini, and bell peppers.

Snack: Hummus with toasted pita chips.

Dinner: Wild rice with dill and lemon roasted salmon fillets.

Wednesday

Breakfast: Cooked quinoa with cinnamon, almond or coconut milk, a spoonful of almond butter, and fruit.

Lunch: Whole-grain tuna fish sandwich with sun-dried tomatoes, Kalamata olives, red onion, capers, olive oil mayonnaise, and lettuce.

Snack: Greek yoghurt with peanut butter, banana, honey, and wheat germ.

Dinner: Pasta with basil and pine nut pesto and roasted chicken.

Thursday

Breakfast: Whole-grain toast topped with avocado, Kalamata olives, sun-dried tomatoes, and pine nuts.

Lunch: Wild rice sautéed with onion, garlic, spinach, basil, and tomatoes and topped with a couple of cooked eggs.

Snack: Roasted eggplant dip with yoghurt, tahini paste, garlic, tomato, and cucumber, with toasted pita chips for dipping.

Dinner: Vegetable stew with lentils, carrots, fire roasted canned tomatoes, vegetable broth, onion, kale, garlic, cumin, and thyme.

Friday

Breakfast: Greek yoghurt topped with honey, almonds, and pomegranate.

Lunch: Whole-wheat orzo with Kalamata olives, tomatoes, spinach, pine nuts, parsley, basil, oregano, garlic, olive oil, and roasted salmon.

Snack: Flatbread topped with thinly sliced and sautéed onions, tomatoes, garlic, and golden beets.

Dinner: Greek Avgolemono soup with chicken, chicken broth, lemon, orzo, and eggs.

Saturday

Breakfast: Oatmeal cooked with apples, chia seeds, cinnamon, and drizzles of both honey and olive oil.

Lunch: Whole-grain pita bread filled with hummus, bean sprouts, cucumber, tomato, olives, feta, and red onion.

Snack: Roasted crispy chickpeas with olive oil, garlic powder, oregano, and lemon juice.

Dinner: Fish tacos with corn tortillas, cod fillets, corn, and cabbage vinaigrette slaw.

Week Two

Sunday

Breakfast: Sweet potato hash with apples, onion, turkey, and poultry seasoning.

Lunch: Salad with lettuce, Kalamata olives, red onion, tomatoes, cucumber, pepperoncini, olive oil based vinaigrette, and topped with salmon.

Snack: Baked root vegetable chips such as beets, carrots, sweet potatoes, and white potatoes dipped in hummus.

Dinner: Red peppers stuffed and roasted with quinoa, sliced cherry tomatoes, basil, parsley, pine nuts, garlic, and red onion.

Monday

Breakfast: Frittata filled with tomatoes, spinach, mushrooms, and feta cheese.

Lunch: Bowl filled with hummus, falafel, Kalamata olives, tomatoes, cucumber, lemon, parsley, and sauce Tzatziki.

Snack: Portobello mushrooms caps filled with fresh mozzarella, basil, and tomatoes and then roasted.

Dinner: Bowtie pasta with sautéed kale, garlic, onion, and pine nuts.

Tuesday

Breakfast: Granola made with oats, almonds, golden raisins, honey, olive oil, cinnamon, and orange zest served with yoghurt or coconut milk.

Lunch: Pasta salad tossed with olive oil, Kalamata olives, tomatoes, cucumber, parsley, basil, kale, Parmesan cheese, and lemon juice.

Snack: Red lentil dip made with cooked red lentils, onion powder, curry powder, garam masala, olive oil, and turmeric served with toasted pita chips.

Dinner: Cooked farro with chickpeas, red onion, garlic, tomatoes, parsley, olive oil, balsamic vinegar, and topped with herb roasted salmon.

Wednesday

Breakfast: Whole grain toast topped with ricotta cheese, figs, honey, and pistachios.

Lunch: Quinoa salad with olive oil, red onion, sun-dried tomato, garlic, lemon, pine nuts, basil, spinach, and Kalamata olives.

Snack: Lavish bread filled with hummus, cucumbers, olives, roasted red peppers, tomatoes, and parsley.

Dinner: Vegetable stew with lentils, carrots, fire roasted canned tomatoes, vegetable broth, onion, kale, garlic, cumin, and thyme.

Thursday

Breakfast: Hummus breakfast bowl with your favorite hummus topped with avocado, lemon juice, and cooked brown rice or quinoa, asparagus, kale, shredded Brussels sprouts, and poached or soft-boiled boiled eggs.

Lunch: Quesadilla filled with spinach, Kalamata olives, sun-dried tomatoes, garlic, mozzarella cheese, feta cheese, and served with Tzatziki sauce.

Snack: Antipasto skewers made with artichoke hearts, fresh mozzarella, olives, cherry tomatoes, roasted red peppers, pepperoncini, and fresh basil.

Dinner: Chicken roasted with potatoes, tomatoes, capers, red peppers, garlic, oregano, parsley, and thyme.

Friday

Breakfast: Chia pudding made by combining chia seeds, coconut milk, a slight bit of honey, cinnamon, and vanilla. Serve the chia pudding with berries or other fruit of choice.

Lunch: Wild rice tossed with lemon, garlic, oregano, and sautéed onion and served topped with roasted chicken.

Snack: Bean salad with cooked beans from fifteen bean soup mix, corn, cherry tomatoes, red onion, bell pepper, scallions, olive oil, parsley, Dijon mustard, balsamic vinegar, and rice vinegar.

Dinner: Stuffed and roasted eggplant with wild rice, tomatoes, Parmesan, lemon, peppers, and white or red onion.

Saturday

Breakfast: Omelet filled with Kalamata olives, artichoke hearts, spinach, tomatoes, and basil.

Lunch: Cooked farro with feta, sun-dried tomatoes, roasted red peppers, pine nuts, cucumber, parsley, basil, and avocado.

Snack: Sliced cucumber topped with mashed avocado and thinly sliced smoked salmon.

Dinner: Stone-ground yellow grits cooked with Parmesan cheese and garlic, topped with shrimp cooked with onions and tomatoes.

Conclusion

Whether you are hoping to lose weight, gain energy, improve your heart health, lower your blood sugar, or overall improve your health and lessen your risk of developing a disease, the Mediterranean diet can help. This diet is more than simply a fad diet to lose weight—rather, it is a lifestyle that has been eaten throughout the Mediterranean for centuries. Rest assured that this diet is backed by countless years of use and many studies conducted by trusted researchers.

It can be scary starting a new journey, but you can feel secure in knowing that through reading this book, you have been provided with all of the tools you need to succeed. Take your journey one step at a time, and before you know it, the Mediterranean lifestyle will feel natural. You can gain the weight loss and health you have dreamed of—all while eating delicious food!

Description

There are countless diets out there claiming to help people lose weight, gain the body of their dreams, and attain health. The truth is that these diets are simple fads with little science to back them up. Fad diets such as these have people giving up fats, carbs, and a number of other foods or entire food groups. The Western world has been taught that being on a diet means restricting oneself.

However, life doesn't have to be this way. It *shouldn't* be this way. The Mediterranean diet is an answer to these problems. While it may be called a diet, it is an entire *lifestyle*. Unlike fad diets, which have only been around for a short time, the Mediterranean diet is the eating style people throughout Mediterranean countries have lived on for centuries. This lifestyle has been tested and proven through time to be effective and maintainable. Not only that, but numerous studies have been conducted on this way of eating—all of which have found it to be beneficial.

While other books may try to sell you a quick scheme to lose weight, the Mediterranean diet doesn't make false promises. You may not lose weight as quickly as you would with a crash or fad diet, but the weight you lose on the Mediterranean diet will stay off unlike with those other ones. All too often, after quitting an unmaintainable crash diet, a person gains back more weight than they lost and are only left with an added five pounds and a damaged metabolism. The same is not true of the Mediterranean diet. Over time, you will slowly gain the weight loss you hope for—but more importantly, you will gain improved health.

Through this book, you will learn how to easily follow the Mediterranean diet to successfully reach your goals. You can learn the science and history behind the

Mediterranean diet in an easy-to-understand manner—gaining helpful insight into this centuries-long lifestyle.

In this book, you will find:

- The deep and varied history of the Mediterranean diet.

- How Dr. Keys developed the Mediterranean diet plan for better health.

- An in-depth look into the science behind the Mediterranean diet and why it works so well.

- The many health benefits of going Mediterranean—including weight loss, heart health, reduced cancer risk, and more.

- How you can start your weight loss journey on the Mediterranean diet.

- Adopting the Mediterranean diet easily with simple-to-follow steps.

- The Mediterranean food pyramid and the healthy foods it contains.

- Answers to frequently asked questions.

- A two-week menu plan complete with breakfast, lunch, snack, and dinner ideas to get you started.

- *And more...*

www.ingramcontent.com/pod-product-compliance
Lightning Source LLC
Chambersburg PA
CBHW080801300326
41914CB00055B/1016